ACKNOWLEDGMENTS

The unified *Pediatric Nursing: Scope and Standards of Practice* was developed by a work group composed of members from both the National Association of Pediatric Nurse Practitioners and the Society of Pediatric Nurses, in collaboration with the American Nurses Association. It addresses pediatric nursing practice at all levels and in all settings and can be used by clinicians, educators, public, regulators, and legislators.

Joint Scope and Standards Writing Work Group Members

Lynn Mohr, MS, PCNS-BC, CPN *(co-Chair, SPN)*
Advocate Hope Children's Hospital, Oak Lawn, IL
Martha K. Swartz, PhD, RN, CPNP *(co-Chair, NAPNAP)*
Yale University School of Nursing, New Haven, CT
Patricia Clinton, PhD, RN, CPNP, FAANP *(NAPNAP; Ex-Officio)*
University of Iowa College of Nursing, Iowa City, IA
Linda Kollar, MSN, CPNP *(NAPNAP)*
Cincinnati Children's Hospital Medical Center, Cincinnati, OH
Carolyn Jaramillo de Montoya, MSN, CPNP *(NAPNAP ; Ex-Officio)*
University of New Mexico, College of Nursing, Albuquerque, NM
Sandy Mott, PhD, RN, BC *(SPN; Ex-Officio)*
Boston College, William F. Connell School of Nursing, Chestnut Hill, MA
LaDonna Northington, DNS, RN, BC, CCRN *(SPN)*
University of Mississippi, School of Nursing, Jackson, MS
Elizabeth Preze, MSN, CPNP PC/AC *(NAPNAP)*
Children's Memorial Hospital, Chicago, IL
Jo Ann Serota, MSN, RN, CPNP *(NAPNAP; Ex-Officio)*
Ambler Pediatrics, Ambler, PA
Linda Youngstrom, DNSc, RN *(SPN)*
Children's Hospital of Philadelphia, Philadelphia, PA
Joal Hill, JD, MPH, PhD *(Ethics consultant)*
Director of Research Ethics Advocate Healthcare, Park Ridge, IL

Joint Scope and Standards Review Panel Work Group Members

Ruth Bindler, PhD, RNC *(SPN)*
Washington State University, Spokane, WA
Mary Bjorklund, MSN, RN, CPN *(SPN)*
Lonestar College, Kingwood, TX

Kristen Bonner, RN *(SPN)*
Saint Vincent Healthcare, Billings, MT
Nan Gaylord, PhD, RN, CPNP *(NAPNAP)*
University of Tennessee, Knoxville, TN
Eva Gomez, MSN, RN *(SPN)*
Children's Hospital Boston, Boston, MA
Catherine Goodhue, MSN, RN, CPNP *(NAPNAP)*
Childrens Hospital Los Angeles, Los Angeles, CA
Peg Harrison, MS, RN, CPNP *(SPN)*
Pediatric Nursing Certification Board, Gaithersburg, MD
Jean Ivey, DSN, CPNP *(NAPNAP)*
University of Alabama at Birmingham, School of Nursing,
Birmingham, AL
Patricia Jackson Allen, MS, RN, PNP, FAAN *(NAPNAP)*
Yale University School of Nursing, New Haven, CT
Andrea M. Kline, RN, MS, CPNP-AC/PC, FCCM *(NAPNAP)*
Children's Memorial Hospital, Chicago, IL
Anne Longo, MBA, BSN, RN-BC *(SPN)*
Cincinnati Children's Hospital, Cincinnati, OH
Debby Mason, MSN, CNP *(SPN)*
Cincinnati Children's Hospital, Cincinnati, OH
Cherie McCann, MSN, RN, BC, CPN *(SPN)*
Pacific Lutheran University, School of Nursing, Tacoma, WA
Armstrong Atlantic State University, Department of Nursing,
Savannah, GA
Sherry McCoy, MSN, RN, CPNP *(NAPNAP)*
Kaiser Permanente, Garden Grove, CA
Barbara Meeks, MSN, MBA, RN *(SPN)*
MCGHealth Children's Medical Center, Augusta, GA
Melissa Reider-Demer, MSN, CPNP *(NAPNAP)*
Childrens Hospital Los Angeles, Los Angeles, CA
Lizabeth Sumner, RN, BSN, RN *(SPN)*
The Elizabeth Hospice, Escondido, CA
Phyllis Thatcher, RN *(SPN)*
Brenner Children's Hospital, Winston-Salem, NC

Joint Scope and Standards Participating Organizations

American Nurses Association (ANA)
National Association of Pediatric Nurse Practitioners (NAPNAP)
Society of Pediatric Nurses (SPN)

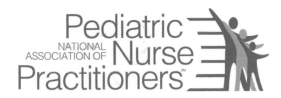

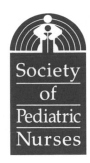

PEDIATRIC NURSING:

SCOPE AND STANDARDS

OF PRACTICE

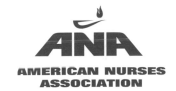

AMERICAN NURSES ASSOCIATION

nurses
books
.org

The Publishing Program of ANA

AMERICAN NURSES ASSOCIATION
SILVER SPRING, MARYLAND
2008

Library of Congress Cataloging-in-Publication data
National Association of Pediatric Nurse Practitioners.

Pediatric nursing : scope and standards of practice / National Association of Pediatric
  Nurse Practitioners, Society of Pediatric Nurses, American Nurses Association.
      p. ; cm.
  Includes bibliographical references and index.
  ISBN-13: 978-1-55810-260-6 (pbk.)
  ISBN-10: 1-55810-260-4 (pbk.)
      1. Pediatric nursing—Standards—United States.   I. Society of Pediatric Nurses.
  II. American Nurses Association. III. Title.
      [DNLM: 1. Pediatric Nursing—standards—Practice Guideline.   2. Clinical
  Competence—Practice Guideline.   3. Nursing Care—standards—Practice Guideline.
  WY 159 N2765p 2008]

  RJ245.N38 2008
      618.92′00231—dc22   2008019887

The American Nurses Association (ANA) is a national professional association. This ANA publication—*Pediatric Nursing: Scope and Standards of Practice*—reflects the thinking of the nursing profession on various issues and should be reviewed in conjunction with state board of nursing policies and practices. State law, rules, and regulations govern the practice of nursing, while *Pediatric Nursing: Scope and Standards of Practice* guides nurses in the application of their professional skills and responsibilities.

Published by Nursesbooks.org
The Publishing Program of ANA

American Nurses Association
8515 Georgia Avenue, Suite 400
Silver Spring, MD 20910-3492
1-800-274-4ANA
http://www.Nursesbooks.org/

ANA is the only full-service professional organization representing the nation's 2.9 million Registered Nurses through its 54 constituent member associations. ANA advances the nursing profession by fostering high standards of nursing practice, promoting the economic and general welfare of nurses in the workplace, projecting a positive and realistic view of nursing, and lobbying the Congress and regulatory agencies on healthcare issues affecting nurses and the public.

Design: Scott Bell, Arlington, VA ~ Freedom by Design, Alexandria, VA ~ Stacy Maguire, Sterling, VA ~ *Copyediting*: Lisa Munsat Anthony, Chapel Hill, NC ~ *Proofreading*: Ashley Mason, Atlanta, GA ~ *Indexing:* Estalita Slivoskey, Ellendale, ND ~ *Composition*: House of Equations, Inc., Arden, NC ~*Printing*: McArdle Printing, Upper Marlboro, MD

First printing June 2008.

ISBN-13: 978-1-55810-260-6   SAN: 851-3481   10M   06/08

American Nurses Association Staff

    Carol J. Bickford, PhD, RN-BC – Content editor
    Yvonne Humes, MLB – Project coordinator
    Maureen Cones – Legal counsel

NAPNAP and SPN Staff

    Dolores C. Jones, EdD, RN, CPNP, CAE *(NAPNAP)*
    Karen KellyThomas, PhD, RN, FAAN, CAE *(NAPNAP)*
    Belinda Puetz, PhD, RN *(SPN)*

About NAPAP

The National Association of Pediatric Nurse Practitioners (NAPNAP) is the professional association for pediatric nurse practitioners and other advanced practice nurses who provide health care for children and families. NAPNAP promotes optimal health for children through leadership, practice, advocacy, education and research. (http://www.napnap.org/)

About SPN

The Society of Pediatric Nurses (SPN) is the premiere pediatric nursing association providing international leadership and promoting the specialty of pediatric nursing in practice, education, and research. The society influences public policy and legislation through collaboration with other nursing organizations and professional organizations dedicated to promoting and improving the health of children. (https://www.pedsnurses.org/)

Descriptions and websites of these groups are in Appendix A, which begins on pg. 85.

CONTENTS

Preface   ix

Introduction   1

    Function of the Scope of Practice Statement   2
    Definition and Function of Standards   2
    Development of Standards   2
    Assumptions   3
    Organizing Principles   3
    Standards of Practice   5
    Standards of Professional Performance   6
    Measurement Criteria   7
    Guidelines   7
    Summary   8

Scope of Pediatric Nursing Practice   9
    Practice Context   9
    Quality and Outcome Guidelines for Nursing of Children   11
      and Families
        Healthcare Home   11
        Family-Centered Care and Management Styles   13
    Evidence-Based Practice   14
    Differentiated Areas of Pediatric Nursing Practice   17
        Pediatric Nurse: Generalist   17
        Advanced Practice Pediatric Nurse   18
            Pediatric Clinical Nurse Specialist (PCNS)   18
            Pediatric Nurse Practitioner (PNP)   19
            Neonatal Nurse Practitioner (NNP)   21
    Settings for Pediatric Nursing Practice   22
        Inpatient and Acute Care Settings   22
        Perioperative and Surgical Settings   22
        Hospice and Palliative Care Settings 23
        Ambulatory Care Settings   23
        Community Health and School Settings 24
        Transport Settings   26
        Camp Settings   26

Caring for a Diverse Population   27
Global Perspectives of Pediatric Nursing   28
Complementary Therapies   28
Education   29
Certification   32
Regulation   33
Professional Issues and Trends   34
Ethical Issues in Pediatric Care   35
Advocacy in Pediatric Care   36
Continued Commitment to the Profession   37

Standards of Pediatric Nursing Practice   **39**

Standards of Practice   **39**
Standard   1. Assessment   39
Standard   2. Diagnosis   43
Standard   3. Outcomes Identification   44
Standard   4. Planning   46
Standard   5. Implementation   47
    Standard 5a. Coordination of Care and Case Management   50
    Standard 5b. Health Teaching and Health Promotion,   51
            Restoration, and Maintenance
    Standard 5c. Consultation   53
    Standard 5d. Prescriptive Authority and Treatment   54
    Standard 5e. Referral   55
Standard   6. Evaluation   56

Standards of Professional Performance   **59**
Standard   7. Quality of Practice   59
Standard   8. Professional Practice Evaluation   61
Standard   9. Education   63
Standard 10. Collegiality   64
Standard 11. Collaboration   65
Standard 12. Ethics   66
Standard 13. Research, Evidence-Based Practice, and   68
            Clinical Scholarship
Standard 14. Resource Utilization   70
Standard 15. Leadership   72
Standard 16. Advocacy   74

References   77

Appendix A: *Scope and Standards of Practice:*   85
              Pediatric Nurse Practitioner (2004)

Appendix B: *Scope and Standards of Pediatric Nursing Practice*   89
              (2003)

Index   171

Preface

Pediatric nursing is the protection, promotion, and optimization of health and abilities for children of newborn age through young adulthood. Utilizing a family-centered care approach, pediatric nursing includes the prevention of illness and injury, the alleviation of suffering through the diagnosis and treatment of the child's response, and advocacy in the care of children and families.

The primary purpose of a scope of practice statement is to protect the public and enhance consumers' access to competent healthcare services. It is also incumbent upon a profession to define the scope and standards of practice within that profession, and to ensure that scope of practice changes reflect the evolution of abilities within the particular healthcare discipline. This publication is the result of a unique, two-year collaborative effort in which members of the National Association of Pediatric Nurse Practitioners (NAPNAP) joined with representatives of the Society of Pediatric Nurses (SPN) and the American Nurses Association (ANA) to launch a new, unified scope and standards of pediatric nursing practice document for the benefit of children, the public, and all the nurses who care for them.

Prior to our efforts, there were two pediatric nursing scope and standards documents available to practitioners, the nursing profession, legislators, regulators, accrediting bodies, and the public. This new publication is based on the ground-breaking work that was put forth in the original *Scope and Standards of Pediatric Nursing Practice* (ANA & SPN, 2003), the *Scope and Standards of Practice: Pediatric Nurse Practitioner (PNP)* (NAPNAP, 2004b) as well as *Nursing: Scope and Standards of Practice* (ANA, 2004). By developing a unified document, NAPNAP and SPN seek to reduce confusion and create a new and improved set of standards that addresses all areas of pediatric nursing practice.

The history of the pediatric specialty within nursing can be traced back to the very early part of the twentieth century. Articles addressing the needs of children appeared in nursing journals as far back as 1906, and the first pediatric nursing text was published in 1923 (Connolly, 2005). General pediatric nursing continued to grow as a specialty throughout the 1900s, and the latter part of the century witnessed the development of professional pediatric nursing organizations, the availability of certification, and the development of standards (Taylor, 2006).

In 1964, Drs. Loretta C. Ford (a pediatric nurse) and Henry K. Silver (a pediatrician) worked together to launch the first PNP program. In that same year, a PNP program was also begun at Massachusetts General Hospital in Boston. The programs' goals were to expand the role of the pediatric nurse to fill gaps in health care for children. The concept was quickly adopted by others, and by 1980 over 300 PNP programs existed (Murphy, 1990). In 1973, the National Association of Pediatric Nurse Associates and Practitioners was formed. (The word "associates" was later dropped from the official NAPNAP name.) Since its inception, NAPNAP has been a leader in many areas for PNPs including education, research, professional development, advocacy, and practice.

SPN was founded in the mid-1980s as a more broad-based pediatric nursing organization whose members now include staff nurses, school and outpatient nurses, clinical nurse specialists, practitioners, administrators, educators, and researchers (Miles, 1996). The Society offers its members the opportunity to interact with colleagues of similar interests and to share ideas, research, and expertise. Through collaborative efforts with other nursing, medical, child health, and child health advocacy groups, the Society also influences legislation, health policy, and public education.

With the evident commonalities in the missions, goals, and activities of both NAPNAP and SPN, it became clear that for both organizations to collaborate and undertake the development of a comprehensive scope and standards document for pediatric nursing would be of benefit to pediatric nurses in all areas of practice, and also provide a unified voice to the public.

In our writing, we were also guided by several assumptions recently described in the monograph *Changes in Healthcare Professions' Scope of Practice: Legislative Consideration* (Association of Social Work Boards et al., 2007). This work, put forth by an interdisciplinary panel of health professional groups (including nursing, social work, medicine, pharmacy, and physical and occupational therapy) suggests the following:

(1) public protection should have top priority in scope of practice decisions;

(2) changes in scope of practice are inherent in our current healthcare system;

(3) collaboration among healthcare providers should be the professional norm; and

(4) overlap among professions is necessary.

That is: no one profession owns a skill or activity in and of itself. Rather, it is the entire scope of activities within a practice that makes a particular profession unique.

Pediatric Nursing: Scope and Standards of Practice describes the scope of activities inherent in pediatric nursing. It describes aspects of competent nursing care and professional performance which are measurable, can be evaluated, and are common to nurses engaged in the care of children and their families based on their generalist or advanced practice role. This one document speaks to the standards of professional performance in all areas of pediatric nursing practice and will serve as a resource not only for nursing faculty and students but also for healthcare providers, researchers, and those involved in funding, legal, policy, and regulatory activities.

We are optimistic that you will find *Pediatric Nursing: Scope and Standards of Practice* useful to you, not only in your daily practice but also when answering larger questions relating to education, public policy and advocacy. We also hope this document will reinforce the inclusion of pediatric nursing as an important component in the plans of study for generalist nurses. The health of our nation's children is dependent on well-educated, qualified, and competent nurses who have the requisite knowledge and skill to care for our more than 71 million children and adolescents living in the United States today.

It took a large team to develop this unified voice. In particular, we would like to acknowledge other members of the writing work group: Linda Kollar and Elizabeth Preze of NAPNAP, and LaDonna Northington, Linda Youngstrom, Sandy Mott, and Belinda Puetz of SPN. Thanks also to Carolyn Jaramillo de Montoya, Patricia Clinton, Jo Ann Serota, Karen KellyThomas, Dolores Jones, and Jennifer Knorr at NAPNAP. After our initial writing, a draft was sent to a Review Panel Work Group consisting of members of both NAPNAP and SPN. Following this, a draft was posted on the ANA, NAPNAP, and SPN web sites for public comment. To all who participated in these important steps, thank you!

In many ways, the work of writing pediatric nursing's scope and standards of practice is an ongoing process, as our profession continues to evolve and the healthcare climate changes. Your input will be invaluable, and we encourage you to be an active part of this process when, in a few short years, we will have another opportunity to update our scope and standards of practice.

Lynn Mohr, MS, RN PCNS-BC CPN (Co-chair, SPN
Martha K. Swartz, PhD, RN, CPNP (Co-chair, NAPNAP)

INTRODUCTION

Pediatric nursing is the protection, promotion, and optimization of health and abilities for children of newborn age through young adulthood. Utilizing a family-centered care approach, pediatric nursing includes the prevention of illness and injury, the alleviation of suffering through the diagnosis and treatment of the child's response, and advocacy in the care of children and families.

Pediatric Nursing: Scope and Standards of Practice is intended to be used in conjunction with *Nursing: Scope and Standards of Practice* (ANA, 2004), *Nursing's Social Policy Statement* (ANA, 2003), *Code of Ethics for Nurses with Interpretive Statements* (ANA, 2001), *Domains and Core Competencies of Nurse Practitioner Practice* (National Organization of Nurse Practitioner Faculties, 2006a), and other documents that outline the values, beliefs, and practice patterns of pediatric nurses. *Pediatric Nursing: Scope and Standards of Practice* reflects and guides the practice of nurses in generalist and advanced practice roles who provide clinical care to children and their families. It may also provide useful information to families and stakeholders such as administrators, educators, policy makers, and others invested in accessing, delivering, and financing health care. Additionally, the document will provide guidance in evaluating the effectiveness and appropriateness of healthcare delivery in pediatric settings.

The National Association of Pediatric Nurse Practitioners (NAPNAP) broadly defines the pediatric population as including all children from birth through 21 years of age, and in specific situations to individuals older than 21 years until appropriate transition to adult health care is successful (NAPNAP, 2002a). There are a growing number of adolescents and young adults with special healthcare needs, chronic conditions, and disabilities who need transition care from pediatric to adult healthcare settings (Betz, 2003, 2004a, & 2004b). With an extensive knowledge base regarding developmental issues and concerns of adolescents and young adults, pediatric nurses are qualified to assist youth during the transition phase. To create an exclusive upper age limit for pediatric patients may unnecessarily create barriers and limit access to health care for this population.

Function of the Scope of Practice Statement

A scope of practice statement describes the *who, what, where, when, why,* and *how* of nursing practice. Each of these questions must be sufficiently answered to provide a complete picture of the practice, its boundaries, and membership. The depth and breadth in which individual nurses engage in the total scope of nursing practice is dependent upon education, certification, individual states' nursing rules and regulations, experience, role, and the population served.

Definition and Function of Standards

Standards are authoritative statements in which the nursing profession describes the responsibilities for which its practitioners are accountable. Consequently, standards reflect the values and priorities of the profession. Standards provide direction for professional nursing practice and a framework for the evaluation of practice. Written in measurable terms, standards also define the nursing profession's accountability to the public and the practice outcomes for which nurses are responsible.

Development of Standards

Standards of professional nursing practice may pertain to general or specialty practice. Each professional nursing organization has a responsibility to its membership and the public it serves to develop standards of practice. This publication is the result of a joint collaboration between the National Association of Pediatric Nurse Practitioners (NAPNAP) and the Society of Pediatric Nurses (SPN). It sets forth standards of pediatric nursing practice and applies them to all nurses engaged in the care of children and their families across care settings. It is based on the original *Scope and Standards of Pediatric Nursing Practice* (ANA & SPN, 2003), *Scope and Standards of Practice: Pediatric Nurse Practitioner (PNP)* (NAPNAP, 2004b) and *Nursing: Scope and Standards of Practice* (ANA, 2004). This document describes aspects of competent nursing care and professional performance which are measurable, can be evaluated, and are common to nurses engaged in the care of children and their families based on their generalist or advanced practice role.

Assumptions

Pediatric Nursing: Scope and Standards of Practice focuses primarily on the processes of providing pediatric nursing care at the generalist and advanced practice levels, and the performance of professional role activities. These standards apply to all nurses involved in the care of children and their families, and they are applicable despite the extensive variability among practice settings. Recognizing the link between the professional work environment and the pediatric nurse's ability to deliver care, employers must provide an environment supportive of nursing practice.

The first major assumption underlying this document is that nursing care is individualized to meet a particular child's or family's unique needs and situation, while focusing on individual, cultural, ethnic, and religious values and beliefs. This includes respect for the goals and preferences of the child and family in developing and implementing a plan of care. Given that one of the nurse's primary responsibilities is need-based patient education, pediatric nurses provide children and their families with individualized information, which empowers children and their families to make informed decisions regarding their health care, including health promotion, prevention of disease, and attainment of a peaceful death.

A second major assumption is that the pediatric nurse establishes a partnership with the child, family, and other healthcare providers. In this partnership, the nurse works collaboratively to coordinate care provided to the child and family. The degree of participation by the child and family will vary based upon preference and ability, and In the case of the child, upon age, developmental abilities, and cognitive understanding of the plan of care.

Organizing Principles

According to *Nursing's Social Policy Statement* (ANA 2003), the recipients of nursing care are individuals, groups, families, communities, and populations. *Pediatric Nursing: Scope and Standards of Practice* uses the terms "client," "patient," "child," and "family" to indicate the person(s) for whom the nurse is providing health care. Care is provided to assist the child or family, sick or well, in performance of those activities contributing to health or its recovery (or to peaceful death), and a return to independence that the child or family would perform unaided if they had the necessary skills, strength, will or knowledge (Alexander et al., 1998; Henderson, 1964).

Consideration of the cultural, racial, ethnic, social, economic, and developmental aspects of the child and family is essential to the provision of nursing services and for developing a plan of care. Precise descriptions of children's health status require viewing children and youth within the context of their environment and development continuum (World Health Organization [WHO] 2007). The *International Classification of Functioning, Disability and Health—Children and Youth Version (ICF–CY)*, which applies classification codes to hundreds of bodily functions and structures, activities, and participation, and various environmental factors that restrict or allow young people to function in an array of everyday activities, enables the accurate and constructive description of children's health (WHO, 2007). Additionally, clients with developmental disabilities are present in all communities and care settings, remaining a vulnerable population. Whatever their age, they and their families need assurance of safe and effective nursing care (Nehring et al. , 2004).

Pediatric Nursing: Scope and Standards of Practice addresses the scope of practice for pediatric nursing which applies to all registered nurses engaged in the nursing care of children and their families, regardless of clinical specialty, practice setting, or educational preparation. Standards that further define the responsibilities of nurses working with children and families in advanced practice roles are also articulated in this document.

Pediatric Nursing: Scope and Standards of Practice provides 16 standards that are categorized as standards of practice and standards of professional performance:

Standards of Practice
1. Assessment
2. Diagnosis
3. Outcomes Identification
4. Planning
5. Implementation

5a. Coordination of Care and Case Management

5b. Health Teaching and Health Promotion, Restoration, and Maintenance

5c. Consultation

5d. Prescriptive Authority and Treatment

5e. Referral

6. Evaluation

Standards of Professional Performance

7. Quality of Practice

8. Professional Practice Evaluation

9. Education

10. Collegiality

11. Ethics

12. Collaboration

13. Research, Evidence-Based Practice, and Clinical Scholarship

14. Resource Utilization

15. Leadership

16. Advocacy

Each category of standards is described below:

Standards of Practice

The six standards of practice describe a competent level of nursing care, as demonstrated by the nursing process, including assessment, diagnosis, outcome identification, planning, implementation, and evaluation. The nursing process encompasses all significant actions taken by nurses in providing care to all patients and families, and it forms the foundation for clinical decision-making and the integration of best research evidence with clinical expertise and patient values (Sackett, Straus, Richardson, Rosenberg, & Haynes 2000). Several themes are common to all areas of nursing practice and reflect nursing responsibilities for all children and their families. These themes merit additional attention and include:

- Providing age-appropriate and culturally and ethnically sensitive care

- Maintaining a safe environment

- Educating children and their families about health practices and treatment modalities

- Providing care that is family-centered as well as efficient, respectful of time, and fiscally responsible

- Ensuring continuity of care

- Coordinating care across settings and among caregivers

- Managing and protecting information

- Communicating effectively inter-professionally and within nursing, as well as in nurse–child–parent interactions

- Ensuring the implementation of evidence-based clinical findings in the practice setting

These themes will be reflected in the measurement criteria associated with various standards in this document, although the wording may be different. They are highlighted here because they are fundamental to many of the standards, and because they have emerged as being consistently and significantly influential in nursing practice today.

Standards of Professional Performance

The ten standards of professional performance describe a competent level of behavior in the professional role, including activities related to quality of care, performance appraisal, outcomes measurement, education, collegiality, ethics, collaboration, research and clinical scholarship, resource utilization, leadership, professional accountability, and advocacy. Within these standards, the advanced practice nurse is expected to be accountable for several other responsibilities that comprise the hallmarks of the profession as well as the advanced practice role. These activities include serving in leadership positions within professional organizations, serving as a role model or mentor to other pediatric nurses, participating in family-centered research, and using evidence-based practice processes to ensure a practice based on evidence. All nurses are expected to engage in professional role activities appropriate to their education, position, and practice setting. Ultimately, nurses are accountable to themselves, patients, and peers for their professional actions.

Measurement Criteria

Pediatric Nursing: Scope and Standards of Practice includes criteria that allow the standards to be measured. These criteria include key indicators of competent practice. To achieve the standards of practice, all criteria must be met, with additional criteria for the advanced practice nurse. Standards should remain stable over time, as they reflect the philosophical values of the profession. However, criteria may be revised to incorporate advancements in scientific knowledge and clinical practice, consultations with other healthcare professionals, and individualized family needs. Criteria must also remain consistent with current nursing practice, education, and research.

Throughout this document, terms such as "appropriate," "pertinent," and "realistic" are used. This document cannot account for all possible scenarios that the pediatric nurse might encounter in clinical practice. The pediatric nurse will need to exercise judgment based on education and experience in determining what is appropriate, pertinent, or realistic. Further direction may be available from documents such as guidelines for practice or agency standards, policies, procedures, protocols, and literature reviews.

Guidelines

Guidelines describe a process of patient care management that has the potential for improving the quality of clinical and consumer decision-making. As systematically developed statements based on available scientific evidence, clinical expertise, and expert opinion, guidelines address the care of specific patient populations or phenomena, whereas standards provide a broad framework for practice. Many practice guidelines have been developed by professional organizations that are applicable to the pediatric population. Guidelines may be used to provide direction for clinical practice policies, procedures, and protocols.

Summary

Pediatric Nursing: Scope and Standards of Practice delineates the professional responsibilities of registered (including advanced practice) nurses engaged in clinical practice related to children and their families, regardless of setting. *Pediatric Nursing: Scope and Standards of Practice* and other nursing practice guidelines serve as a basis for:

- Quality improvement systems
- Data system development
- Regulatory systems
- Healthcare reimbursement and financing methodologies
- Development and evaluation of nursing service delivery systems and organizational structures
- Certification activities
- Job descriptions and performance appraisals
- Agency policies, procedures, and protocols
- Educational offerings
- Research activities
- Consistency in care
- Professional development
- Global health

In order to best serve the public and the nursing profession, pediatric nurses must continue to contribute to the development of standards of practice and evidence-based practice guidelines. Nursing must examine how standards and practice guidelines can be disseminated and used more effectively to enhance and promote the quality of clinical practice. In addition, standards and practice guidelines must be evaluated on an ongoing basis, with revisions made as necessary. The dynamic nature of the healthcare environment and the growing body of nursing research provide both the impetus and the opportunity for nursing to ensure competent clinical practice and to promote ongoing professional development that enhances the quality of pediatric nursing care.

Scope of Pediatric Nursing Practice

The scope of practice and roles of the pediatric nurse are diverse and dynamic. The intention of this document is to identify some of the issues and trends that define current roles and to highlight the variety of pediatric nursing roles that have evolved to meet the ever-changing healthcare needs of children and their families in a variety of settings. The document is not intended to restrict role development, but rather to clarify the scope and foundation of general as well as advanced practice pediatric nursing and to distinguish between these areas of practice.

Practice Context

There are approximately 73 million children and adolescents in the United States, accounting for one-fourth of the nation's population (U.S. Department of Health and Human Services, 2005). Approximately 20% of children experience special healthcare needs, chronic illness, or disability. The most prevalent chronic conditions among children are asthma (affecting 12% of children), learning disabilities (affecting 8%) and attention-deficit hyperactivity disorder (affecting 7%).

For children and adolescents who do not experience a chronic illness or condition, major threats to health include accidents, violence, substance abuse, and sexually transmitted illnesses. Injuries are the leading cause of death among those 1 to 24 years of age, and over 50% of injuries are related to motor vehicle collisions (U.S. Department of Health and Human Services, 2002).

Children, families, and all citizens are significantly affected by the growing problem of youth violence. According to an integrative review (Gance-Cleveland, 2001), youths are three times more likely than adults to be victims of a violent crime, and homicide is the second leading cause of death among youths age 15–24 years. It is estimated that 270,000 guns are taken to school each day in the United States, while firearms in the home also provide a risk for unintentional injury. Overall, the threat of terrorism and bioterrorism places further stress and strain on the ability of children and their families to cope with uncertainty.

In the United States, minorities and the poor experience disparities in access to health care, health-related quality of life, and illness and death.

A recent analysis by the Children's Defense Fund (CDF) of data from the National Health Interview Survey revealed significant racial and ethnic differences of the effects of healthcare coverage and income on outcomes (CDF, 2006). Among the findings by the CDF are:

- Latino children are almost three times as likely and African–American children are almost twice as likely as Caucasian children to be uninsured;

- among the uninsured, African–American children are 60% more likely than Caucasian children to have an unmet healthcare need; and

- similar percentages of African–American and Caucasian low-income children have gone two or more years without receiving dental care and have experienced limitations due to a chronic illness or disability.

The findings of the CDF further indicate that among children, disparities persist in the rates of infant mortality, immunizations, asthma, lead poisoning, and obesity. These are conditions that may impact many aspects of a child's health and development and can have lasting effects throughout adolescence and into adulthood. Because childhood is a time of physical, social, intellectual, and emotional growth, pediatric nursing practice must be aimed at the prevention, early identification, and intervention for health problems that may extend to adulthood. To reduce healthcare disparities, pediatric nurses advocate for and provide quality health care. Additionally, they work with the community and policy makers to foster awareness of child health disparities, and they may work with other clinicians and public health officials in coalitions to identify resources, and implement and evaluate programs of health care.

To further explore the effect of recent governmental programs on children's access to health care, a pediatric nurse practitioner (PNP) headed an evaluative study of the State Child Health Insurance Program (SCHIP), published in *Pediatrics* (Duderstadt, Hughes, Soobader & Newacheck, 2006). Like the CDF, Duderstadt and colleagues also analyzed data comparing the 1997 and 2003 National Health Interview Survey. Findings revealed that children in the SCHIP target income group experienced the largest reduction in rates of uninsurance, and the percentage of children without a usual source of care or a primary care provider was also reduced. However, the implementation of the SCHIP program led to no significant changes in the level of reported unmet needs, volume of provider visits, receipt of well-child care, and dental care. Thus, while the SCHIP program has increased the rates of Medicaid enrollment for children in eligible families, healthcare disparities persist. Pediatric nurses are key to advocating for families, making policy recommendations, and evaluating the effects of such programs through research and education.

Quality and Outcome Guidelines for Nursing of Children and Families

Beginning in 2001, the Expert Panel on Children and Families of the American Academy of Nursing initiated a collaborative process to identify the key standards of excellence in the nursing of children and families (Craft-Rosenberg & Krajicek, 2006). These guidelines were developed by a coalition of pediatric and family nurses representing 12 professional organizations, including SPN and NAPNAP. The 18 guidelines of this "paradigm of excellence" provide a template for clinicians, educators, researchers, and policy makers to promote, evaluate, and improve the quality of health care that is provided to children and families (Table 1).

The recently published text *Nursing Excellence for Children and Families* devotes a chapter to each of the guidelines, with each chapter presenting a review and analysis of the evidence pertaining to the guideline as well as implications for practice (Craft-Rosenberg & Krajicek, 2006). Clinicians may apply the guidelines to evaluate and change nursing care in the clinical setting. They may also be used by educators for curriculum revision and by researchers as a framework for testing interventions to evaluate effectiveness and outcomes. A consumer version of the guidelines has also been developed so that patients and families may evaluate the quality of care received.

Healthcare Home

The concept *healthcare home* or *medical home* provides a framework to improve access to care and eliminate disparities in health (including dental) care for children and families through effective care coordination and case management (Cowell & Swartwout, 2006). NAPNAP advocates for a pediatric healthcare home that is "accessible, comprehensive, coordinated, culturally sensitive and focused on the overall well-being

T A B L E 1 Healthcare Quality and Outcome Guidelines

1. Children and youth have an identified healthcare home.
2. The families of children and youth are partners in decisions, planning, and delivery of care.
3. Family values, beliefs, and preferences are part of care.
4. Family strengths and main concerns are obvious in the care of children and youth.
5. Children, youth, and families will have accessible health care.
6. Pregnant women will have accessible health care.
7. Family needs are identified and services are offered.
8. Children, youth, and families are directed to community services when needed.
9. Children, youth, and families receive care that promotes and maintains health and prevents disease.
10. Pregnant women, children, youth, and families have access to genetic testing and advice.
11. Children and youth receive care that is physically and emotionally safe.
12. Children's, youth's, and families' privacy and rights are protected.
13. Children and youth who are very ill receive the full range of needed services.
14. Children and youth with disabilities and/or special healthcare needs receive the full range of services.
15. Children, youth, and families receive comfort care.
16. Children's, youths', and families' health and risky behaviors and problems are identified and addressed.
17. Children, youth, and families receive care that supports development.
18. Children, youth, and families are fully informed of the outcomes of care.

From Craft-Rosenberg, M. & Krajicek, M. (2006). *Nursing excellence for children and families.* New York, NY: Springer Publishing Co.

of the child within the family" (NAPNAP, 2002b). NAPNAP further asserts that all children should have access to comprehensive health care by their pediatric healthcare professional of choice, and that all healthcare providers, including pediatricians, pediatric subspecialists, pediatric nurse practitioners, nurses, and clinical nurse specialists, should have a collaborative role in the provision of such care. Such care should be available without barriers to service resulting from financial or insurance restrictions, lack of available providers, or other difficulties (NAPNAP, 2007).

While *healthcare home* or *medical home* is a relatively new label, the elements of such care can historically be traced back to public health nursing and the community mental health movement which provided guidelines for providing care to the underserved (APHA, 1955; Caplan, 1961; Pridham, 1993). Nursing has continued to be a driving force in the development of innovative models for providing high quality health care including school-based health centers (SBHCs) and community health centers. Because nurses interact with consumers at multiple entry points in the healthcare system, they play a key role in implementing the healthcare home concept and assuring that care is accessible, comprehensive, continuous, and culturally competent. According to Cowell & Swartwout (2006), nursing care excellence in implementing the healthcare home concept is achieved by:

- supporting the delivery of care via interdisciplinary teams;
- creating effective communication and partnerships with each family;
- enabling a central location for healthcare records;
- involving family members and individualizing care;
- being an expert at knowing community resources;
- being an expert on state and federal policies, regulations, and programs;
- implementing a quality monitoring system;
- promoting and monitoring preventive care;
- providing comprehensive primary care;
- providing creative solutions for those who are uninsured;
- providing support during periods of transition;
- working with families with special needs;
- assisting families in becoming independent, informed consumers of health care; and
- generating nursing research related to the healthcare home concept.

Family-Centered Care and Management Styles

Family-Centered Care is a philosophy of care that acknowledges the importance of family partnerships in nursing care whereby the family is an active partner or collaborator in the process, not a passive recipient of the professional's expertise (Deatrick, 2006). With an increase in the number of single-parent and blended families, traditional definitions of family that are grounded in biological ties are no longer useful. Shelton and Stepanek (1994) maintain that the first step in providing Family-Centered Care is to understand how a family defines itself and who the child considers as family members.

The Family-Centered Care model recognizes the family as the constant in the child's life and central in the child's plan of care. Eight elements of Family-Centered Care have been defined, each serving to reinforce, facilitate, and complement the implementation of the others (see Table 2). These elements recognize each family's uniqueness, acknowledge the influence of the family as a constant in the child's life, and emphasize the importance of providing health care which reflects the value of collaboration between the child, family, and the healthcare team. Family-Centered Care is based upon the premise that a positive adjustment to a child's level of health and well-being requires the involvement of the whole family. *Family-Centered Care: Putting it into Action—The SPN/ANA Guide to Family-Centered Care* further expands upon these elements and provides evidence-based practice recommendations that more fully describe this model (Lewandowski & Tesler, 2003).

In order to build partnerships with families, nurses and healthcare providers need standardized guidelines and descriptions of family coping styles in order to individualize their approaches to families. The Family Management Style (FMS) framework was developed over a 20-year period through reviews of qualitative research and concept development. Five family management styles or patterns describing how families define and manage illness-related demands and the resulting consequences for family life have emerged: thriving, accommodating, enduring, struggling, and floundering (Deatrick & Knafl, 1990; Knafl, Breitmayer, Gallo & Zoeller 1996; Knafl & Deatrick 2002). The styles represent the continuum of difficulties that families experience when managing a child's illness and also provide a basis for individualized care planning.

Evidence-based Practice

There is concern among healthcare organizations, federal agencies, and the public regarding the large time gap between the publication of

T A B L E 2 Key Elements of Family-Centered Care

Element 1: The Family at the Center

Incorporate into policy and practice the recognition that family is the constant in a child's life, while the service systems and support personnel within those systems fluctuate and that the illness or injury of a child affects all members of the family.

Element 2: Family–Professional Collaboration

Facilitate family-professional collaboration at all levels of hospital, home, and community care for:
- Care of an individual child;
- Program development, implementation, evaluation and evolution;
- Policy formation.

Element 3: Family-Professional Communication

Exchange complete and unbiased information between families and professionals in a supportive manner at all times.

Element 4: Cultural Diversity of the Family

Incorporate into policy and practice the recognition and of honoring of cultural diversity, strengths, and individuality within and across all families, including ethnic,racial, spiritual, social, economic, educational, and geographic diversity.

Element 5: Coping Differences and Supports

Recognize and respect different methods of coping and implement comprehensive policies and programs that provide families with the developmental, educational, emotional, spiritual, environmental, and financial supports needed to meet their diverse needs.

Element 6: Family-Centered Peer Support

Encourage and facilitate family-to-family support networking.

Element 7: Specialized Service and Support Systems

Ensure that hospital, home, and community service and support systems for children needing specialized health and developmental care and their families are flexible, accessible, and comprehensive in responding to diverse family-identified needs.

Element 8: Holistic Perspective of Family-Centered Care

Appreciate families as families and children as children, recognizing that they possess a wide range of strengths, concerns emotions and aspirations beyond their need for specialized health and developmental services and support.

From Lewandowski, L. & Tesler, M. (2003). *Family-Centered Care: Putting it Into Action – The SPN/ANA Guide to Family-Centered Care.* Washington, DC: Nursebooks.org.

research findings and the translation of findings into practice to improve patient care. Furthermore, the findings reported by the Institute of Medicine (2001) in *Crossing the Quality Chasm: A New Health System for the 21st Century* have challenged all healthcare professionals to deliver care that is based upon the best scientific evidence available. Evidence-based practice (EBP) has been defined as "the integration of best research evidence with clinical expertise and patient values" (Sackett, Straus, Richardson, Rosenberg & Haynes, 2000). In nursing, several evidence-based nursing centers have been developed at leading universities (Brady & Lewin, 2007).

Increasingly, clinical practice guidelines are being developed by professional organizations or expert panels that promote the translation of evidence-based findings into nursing care (Melnyk & Fineout-Overholt, 2005). One such example is the *Healthy Eating and Activity Together (HEAT^SM) Clinical Practice Guideline: Identifying and Preventing Overweight in Childhood*, published by NAPNAP (2006b), which is aimed at the prevention of overweight and obesity in children. A key component of this guideline is the inclusion of culturally appropriate strategies for groups most at risk for childhood overweight (Hispanics, African–Americans, and Native Americans).

Similarly, NAPNAP has also developed the national program *KySS^SM: Keep Your Children/Yourself Safe and Secure*, and a supporting *The KySS^SM Guide to Child and Adolescent Mental Health Screening, Early Intervention and Health Promotion* (Melnyk & Moldenhauer, 2006) which is geared toward the prevention and subsequent decrease of psychosocial morbidities in children and teenagers. The program emphasizes educational–behavioral interventions to teach children, youth, and their parents all aspects of physical and emotional safety, and to build self-esteem, and to strengthen other developmental assets such as positive coping and problem-solving skills.

Pediatric nurses acknowledge the need for evidence-based practice in the clinical setting and recognize that continuing research, including research involving children, will be required to gather that evidence. Pediatric nurses advocate for research where minimal risk to the child is involved and potential benefits outweigh risks. Pediatric nurses promote research that is conducted in a respectful, ethical manner in the hope that findings will benefit the children involved in the studies and the future care of children (NAPNAP, 2004a; SPN, 2004).

Differentiated Areas of Pediatric Nursing Practice

Pediatric nurses are licensed registered nurses who provide health care to children through either a generalist or advanced practice role. These areas of practice are described below.

Pediatric Nurse: Generalist

The pediatric nurse who practices as a *generalist* is a licensed registered nurse who has demonstrated clinical skills and knowledge within the specialty. Many nurses who contribute to the care of children and their families are also responsible for adhering to the specialty practice standards as designated by the profession.

In 1998, SPN completed a project funded by the Health Resources and Services Administration (HRSA) Maternal and Child Bureau that identified standards for pediatric pre-licensure and early professional development (Woodring & Pridham, 1998). While these concepts and competencies apply to the education of the beginning practitioner, they offer a unique description of the elements of pediatric nursing including:

- the unique anatomical, physiological, and developmental differences among neonates, infants, children, adolescents, and young adults in transition;
- care of children in the context of their families;
- sensitivity to cultural issues, especially those related to how the family and healthcare providers tend to children's healthcare needs;
- effective communication with children, families, other healthcare providers, and appropriate educational agency staff;
- safety assurance and injury prevention for children and their families;
- promotion of children's health in the context of their families;
- assessment of the unique growth and development needs of children who have chronic conditions, and of their families;
- exceptional needs of children with episodic injuries or illnesses;
- economic, social, and political influences outside the family that have an impact on children's health and development and family functioning; and
- ethical, moral, and legal dilemmas involving children, families, and healthcare professionals.

Advanced Practice Pediatric Nurse

Advanced practice registered nurses (APRNs) are registered nurses (RNs) who have acquired advanced education (either a master's or doctoral degree) and have developed specialized clinical knowledge and skills to provide health care. They build upon the practice of RNs by demonstrating a greater depth and breadth of knowledge, a strong ability to synthesize data and employ critical thinking, increased complexity of skills and interventions, and significant role autonomy (ANA, 2004). The APRN role combines both specialization and expansion through in-depth study of the research-based, theoretical, and clinical practice issues unique to the specialty population.

In pediatric nursing, the predominant advanced practice roles are the pediatric clinical nurse specialist (PCNS), the primary care pediatric nurse practitioner (PNP-PC), the acute care pediatric nurse practitioner (PNP-AC), and the neonatal nurse practitioner (NNP). The advanced practice pediatric nurse holds a minimum of a master's degree in pediatric nursing, has attained certification in the advanced practice role, and holds the appropriate credentials as determined by the state Board of Nursing. The pediatric APRN provides care in an expanded role that incorporates comprehensive assessment skills, diagnostic ability, critical thinking, independent decision-making, collaborative management of health and illness problems, leadership within complex systems, and the ability to critically analyze and translate research findings into practice. APRNs in other clinical settings, such as family practice, nurse midwifery, and nurse anesthesia, are also expected to incorporate advanced knowledge of pediatric concepts into their clinical practice to the extent that their client populations may include pediatric patients and their families.

The advanced practice pediatric nursing roles are differentiated from one another by virtue of their unique blend of nursing knowledge, science, and practice settings. The following descriptions further illustrate the advanced practice roles which require knowledge specialization and clinical expertise in the care of children and their families:

Pediatric Clinical Nurse Specialist (PCNS)

The PCNS is an APRN prepared as a clinical expert in the specialty of pediatric nursing and who, in addition to providing direct patient care, serves as a leader in education, research, quality improvement, outcome monitoring, and consultation with other nurses, health team members, and the community. Clinical nurse specialists are prepared at the master's or doctoral level. CNSs are generally employed and paid by a healthcare institution, or they may work independently in private or collaborative practice. The National Association of Clinical Nurse Specialists (NACNS) has published a position statement on CNS education and practice in which they identify core CNS competencies and the corresponding core areas of knowledge that should be included in CNS graduate programs (NACNS 2004). The core areas of knowledge are expanded from the core areas identified in the American Association of Colleges of Nursing's (AACN) *Essentials of Master's Education for Advance Practice Nursing* (1996) document and include theoretical foundations, inquiry skills, empirical and practical knowledge that focus on phenomena of concern, nursing therapeutics, evaluation methodologies, and systems thinking.

Pediatric Nurse Practitioner (PNP)

The PNP provides comprehensive health care to children from birth through young adulthood by assessment, diagnosis, management, and evaluation of care. In accordance with state licensure and regulatory mechanisms, PNPs provide a wide range of pediatric healthcare services in a variety of primary and specialty healthcare settings, with a strong emphasis on health promotion, injury and disease prevention, and management and coping with chronic illness. The PNP may consult with other members of the healthcare team, coordinate care, and make referrals to other healthcare providers. Additionally, the PNP may function as a consultant in areas of expertise to colleagues in health professions and other disciplines. The PNP assumes accountability for professional actions and incorporates risk management strategies into clinical practice. Today, PNPs practice not only in primary care but also in acute and specialty care settings. While the types of settings have expanded, the fundamental aspects and essential components of the PNP remain consistent across settings. There are now two broad categories of PNPs: those who practice predominantly in primary care settings and those who practice in acute care settings.

Historically, PNPs have practiced predominantly in primary care settings in which the emphasis is on providing health care that is accessible, comprehensive in scope, and coordinated with specialty practices and community resources in order to maximize continuity. Certification as a PNP, with an emphasis on primary care, is offered by both the Pediatric Nursing Certification Board (PNCB) and the American Nurses Credentialing Center (ANCC) and is required for recognition in most states.

The acute care PNP provides cost-effective, quality care for acutely, critically, and chronically ill children who may be experiencing life-threatening illnesses and organ dysfunction or failure. Similar to the primary care PNP, direct patient care management by the acute care PNP within a collaborative practice model includes performing in-depth physical assessments, ordering and interpreting results of laboratory and diagnostic tests, ordering medications, and performing therapeutic procedures in a variety of contexts which may include inpatient and outpatient hospital units, emergency departments, and home care settings. The foundation of advanced practice nursing also provides general role expectations for the acute care PNP which include expertise in patient care that is based on clinical evidence and theory, progressive leadership, and involvement in education and research.

The role of the acute care PNP began to evolve in the late 1990s, as nurse practitioner practice expanded into critical care units, specialty practice sites, and emergency departments. The expansion of the role was also in keeping with recommendations of the Institute of Medicine, which called for a greater commitment to interdisciplinary care (2001). The increased demand for PNPs with knowledge and skills necessary for acute care practice led to progressive changes in the education of PNPs for this role. In 2004, NAPNAP developed a position statement for the acute care PNP (NAPNAP, 2005a). Similarly, the National Panel for Acute Care Nurse Practitioner Competencies, in collaboration with the Association of Faculties of PNP Programs (AFPNP), developed a set of core competencies for PNPs in acute care (2004). These competencies now provide the basis for curriculum development, evaluation, and certification. The PNCB offered the first certification examination for the acute care PNP in January 2005 to those who met the standards of review by the PNCB, based on the competencies. Currently, graduation from an acute care PNP program is required to sit for the PNCB acute care PNP examination. As with other nursing roles, the requirements for entry into practice and for recognition of the acute care PNP role vary from state to state. As of this writing, the majority of states (31) require that acute care PNPs take a pediatric acute care certification examination in order to be fully licensed by the state (Percy & Sperhac, 2007).

Neonatal Nurse Practitioner (NNP)

NNPs provide healthcare services to high-risk infants in neonatal intensive care units (NICUs), well baby nurseries, and in follow-up clinics (for children 2 years of age and younger). The NNP services include providing diagnosis and management of neonatal diseases, health promotion, and follow-up care of high-risk babies. NNP competencies have also been developed by the National Association of Neonatal Nurses (NANN) to reflect the educational standards for neonatal nurse practitioner programs (NANN, 2002). The standards are based on a foundation of the broad standards for advanced nursing practice (American Association of Colleges of Nursing 1996) and the evaluation criteria for nurse practitioner programs.

All nurse practitioners and clinical nurse specialists function according to their state Nurse Practice Act and in accordance with individual state laws and regulations. States vary in their regulations, including the granting of prescriptive privileges, and specific state requirements must be recognized and met. In some states, current impediments to the full use of advanced practice nurses include:

(1) legal barriers such as laws that require physician supervision or limit a nurse's prescriptive authority,

(2) financial barriers that prevent public and private payers from reimbursing advanced practice nurses, and

(3) professional barriers.

As Safriet (1992) has stated, "Advanced practice nurses have demonstrated repeatedly that they can provide cost-effective, high quality primary care for many of the neediest members of society, but their role has been severely limited by restrictions on their scope of practice, prescriptive authority, and eligibility for reimbursement" (p. 417). Fortunately, healthcare regulatory organizations now acknowledge that it is not reasonable to expect each health profession to have a completely unique scope of practice, and that there is considerable overlap among the abilities and skill sets of each discipline (Association of Social Work Boards et al, 2007). Scope of practice changes should reflect the evolution of the abilities of practitioners within a healthcare discipline to provide care in a safe and effective manner, in order to better protect the public and enhance consumer access to quality health care.

Settings for Pediatric Nursing Practice

Inpatient and Acute Care Settings

Practice settings for pediatric nursing are multiple and varied. Free-standing children's hospitals, which are solely dedicated to providing acute care and rehabilitation services to the pediatric population, represent just 1% of all hospitals, but account for 39% of all admissions, 49% of inpatient days, and 59% of hospital costs (National Association of Children's Hospitals and Related Institutions, 2001). There are other facilities (e.g., pediatric and adolescent units, pediatric and neonatal intensive care units) where pediatric specialty services are provided within a multi-focused acute care setting. Children's hospitals and major teaching hospitals together treat 98% of all children requiring heart or lung transplants, 88% of all children with cancer needing in-patient care, and 76% of all children hospitalized with cystic fibrosis (National Association of Children's Hospitals and Related Institutions, 2001). In addition, children's hospitals are key providers for the 35% of children who are either uninsured or dependent on Medicaid and other public sources for payment of health care.

Perioperative and Surgical Settings

The pediatric surgical environment creates an additional setting for pediatric nursing. Pediatric surgical nursing involves care for children throughout the surgical experience, including pre-operative preparation and teaching, intra-operative care in both inpatient and out-patient settings, and post-operative care for major surgery, minimally invasive surgery, innovative therapies, fetal surgery, pediatric solid organ transplantation, surgery for congenital anomalies, and more. Perioperative nurses provide direct patient care, coordinate the multidisciplinary surgical care team, and provide emotional and psychosocial support to the family and child. The American Pediatric Surgical Nurses Association (APSNA) is the specialty organization for those pediatric nurses involved in perioperative nursing.

Hospice and Palliative Care Settings

In the United States, it is estimated that 53,000 children from newborns through 19 years of age die each year, with 75–85% of children dying in the hospital—many in the intensive care setting (Field & Behrman, 2003). Less than 1% of these children die in a pediatric hospice setting.

Palliative care, which can take place in the hospital or home setting, focuses on enhancing the quality of remaining life by assisting the child and family to meet the goals they have set. It is not meant to hasten or postpone death but coexists with curative measures. Care can change as the child advances through the disease process and as death approaches. Palliative care can give dignity to life and allows death to happen in a manner that is meaningful for the family. When families are faced with complex medical or life decisions regarding the care of their child, such as whether to continue or withhold treatment, the pediatric palliative nurse can facilitate patient–family communication, provide specific clinical information, and assist with the palliative care plan.

Hospice care is care provided at the end of life where the disease has been deemed either incurable or terminal with a life expectancy of six months or less. The focus is non-curative treatment with aggressive management of symptoms aimed at improving the quality of life at the end of life and facilitating bereavement once death has occurred. The pediatric hospice nurse assists the family through the dying and bereavement process.

Ambulatory Care Settings

Ambulatory care settings offer children and their families ongoing contact with healthcare professionals. Due to long-term, ongoing contact with the family, the nurse in this setting has an opportunity to develop a mutually gratifying and therapeutic relationship with the child and family. This long-term relationship can provide a more complete picture of the child's general well-being and ability to achieve developmental milestones. Illness prevention and health promotion activities are the core interventions of the nurse and the healthcare team. For children coping with a chronic condition, the healthcare team also focuses on maintaining optimum levels of health for the child.

The nurse practicing in a specialty pediatric clinic collaborates with a multidisciplinary team to meet the challenges of patients with a chronic or terminal illness. Quality health care for these children often requires significant case coordination so that the care provided is accessible, comprehensive, continuous, and efficient. Throughout the care process, the nurse serves as a vital link in the communication between health team members and the family.

Community Health and School Settings

Community health settings provide the pediatric nurse an opportunity to positively affect large populations of children and families through community health organizations, schools, and city and state departments of health. Many community health programs are aimed at prevention, education, and provision of programs (such as immunizations and screening). Pediatric nurses practicing in home health care address the environmental, social, and personal factors affecting health and may provide care that cannot be offered by family or friends on a consistent basis. The focus of home health care is on preventing admission to an acute care setting, providing assistance to families, and providing direct treatment in the home.

Pediatric nurses working in schools may be employed by a local school system (either public or private), or by a county, city, or state governmental agency. The National Association of School Nurses (NASN) developed a resolution paper on the need for access to school nurses and a position statement outlining the need for school nurses in caring for chronically ill children (NASN, 2003, 2006). The school nurse is often responsible for meeting the needs of children in more than one school and ideally works with an aide, health associate, and other unlicensed assistive personnel who are responsible for monitoring day-to-day school health problems. The school nurse is responsible for overall management and delegation of activities to the aides and for evaluating the appropriateness of interventions provided to ailing children.

School nursing is a specialized practice of professional nursing that advances the well-being, academic success, and life-long achievement of students. The educational requirements for school nurses vary from state to state; however, the NASN recommends a baccalaureate degree in nursing from an accredited college or university and licensure as a registered nurse as the minimal preparation for the skills needed for entering school nursing practice (NASN, 2002). School nurses work with the students, parents or guardians, healthcare practitioners, teachers, school administrators, and other professionals in the school setting and the community to provide or secure health services for children.

School nurses need to have expertise in clinical nursing, communication, surveillance, education, advocacy, and leadership in order to ensure that all students' health needs are addressed. The school nurse's role includes assessing the health status of students, identifying health problems that have an impact on health and learning, delivering emergency care, administering medications, performing healthcare procedures, providing wellness programs, advocating for children and families, and providing health counseling and health education. School nurses may be deemed first responders related to infectious disease outbreaks and episodes of violence or bioterrorism within and around the school. Overall, school nursing involves planning, developing, managing, and evaluating healthcare services to children in an educational setting and encompasses working with the families of the students and the community in which the student resides (Guilday, 2000; NASN & ANA, 2005).

School-based health centers (SBHCs) provide comprehensive physical and mental health services to children, with parental involvement, at locations accessible to children. SBHCs are not designed to replace an ongoing relationship a child may have with a primary provider, nor to replace the services of a school nurse. Rather, the SBHCs are designed to overcome existing social and economic barriers that prevent access to quality health care. Ideally, students receive comprehensive primary care, delivered in the context of family and community, which includes social services, mental health, and health education with a focus on wellness so that they may derive maximum benefit from their education (NAPNAP, 2005b). SBHCs should meet standards of care similar to those of community health centers, including certification and credentialing processes and a systematic evaluation of outcomes of services (Gance-Cleveland, Costin, & Degenstein, 2003).

These clinics are usually staffed by a pediatric nurse practitioner or physician's assistant, and a clinic assistant or receptionist, with access to a team of health educators, physicians, nutritionists, nurses, and social workers. The staff is trained to deal with the unique growth, social, developmental, and emotional needs of the school age population they serve. Activities of the school nurse or clinic may also include sponsoring health fairs and immunization programs, ongoing participation in crisis intervention teams, class health education, parent education, teacher training, sports medicine clinics, student health clubs, question-and-answer columns in student newspapers, involvement in dropout prevention initiatives, and assessing health risk behaviors of the student population.

Pediatric nurses also provide health consultation to early care and education (ECE) programs (Crowley, 2001). The role of the child care health consultant (CCHC) is to minimize health risks and promote healthy behaviors in out-of-home care programs, and to link families with community-based health and developmental services (Ramler et al, 2006). Specifically, CCHCs promote health practices in ECE programs that may focus on nutrition, safe food handling, infection control, infant sleep position, monitoring of immunizations, and safe and active play. Evidence is emerging that the role of the CCHC can improve overall child care quality and school readiness among children (Ramler et al., 2006).

Transport Settings

Another setting for pediatric nursing practice is in air and surface transport. Neonates and infants who have increased acute care needs and technological support requirements may need air or surface transport from a community hospital or birth hospital to a facility with tertiary intensive capabilities. Young children and adolescents may require transport to a pediatric intensive care or other subspecialty unit. Pediatric specialty teams are typically composed of two RNs, an RN and NP, an RN and MD, or an RN with an MD and a Respiratory Therapist. The Air and Surface Transport Nurses Association (ASTNA) is a professional association for nurses working in the transport settings.

Camp Settings

Camp nursing affords the pediatric nurse the opportunity to provide all aspects of health care in an outdoor setting to either the general pediatric population or a specialty population (such as children with cancer, cystic fibrosis, asthma, diabetes, or developmental disabilities). The primary goal of the specialty camps is to allow the children, who may have had extensive or unpleasant medical treatment and life experiences, to enjoy a real camping experience while also learning about their illness or disability. Experienced pediatric nurses with current Basic Life Support training and Basic First Aid Training may choose to practice in camp settings. The Association of Camp Nurses has published a *Standards and Scope of Camp Nursing Practice* document (ACN, 2002) available for ordering at http://www.campnurse.org/store/acn.html.

Caring for a Diverse Population

Providing culturally competent care that values diversity, is based on self-assessment, and effectively manages the dynamics of differences between individuals and groups is fundamental to nursing practice. Due to the expanding cultural diversity of the American population, it is imperative that pediatric nurses understand and have a working knowledge of cultural characteristics and practices of the populations most served in their clinical area and are also aware of their own values and prejudices. Understanding cultural views can assist the pediatric nurse to anticipate and understand why and how families make certain decisions regarding their child's health. The pediatric nurse should expect that cultural and religious beliefs and practices may affect the management of the ill child, so these must be incorporated into the child and family care plan. When necessary, however, adjustments may need to be made when beliefs and practices are deemed unsafe for the child. For the pediatric nurse, it is imperative to apply knowledge of and demonstrate respect for culture and religion as a framework in the provision of care.

An appreciation of diversity and the promotion of inclusivity are also important when providing care to youth who are or think they may be gay, lesbian, bisexual, transgender, or who are struggling with or questioning their sexual orientation or gender identity (gay, lesbian, bisexual, transgender, and questioning; GLBTQ). Many GLBTQ youth are exposed to prejudice and encounter stigma, hostility or hatred which may hinder their ability to achieve developmental tasks (Harrison, 2003). These children tend to experience higher levels of isolation, runaway behavior, homelessness, domestic violence, depression, anxiety, suicide, violent victimization, substance abuse, and school or job failure as compared with heterosexual or gender-conforming youth (Nelson, 2003). Pediatric nurses should individualize interventions relating to health promotion and risk reduction for youth who identify or who are struggling whether to identify themselves as GLBTQ (NAPNAP, 2006a).

Global Perspectives of Pediatric Nursing

With the increasing ease at which people can travel worldwide, many opportunities exist for pediatric nursing globally. Many nurses travel to underdeveloped countries as part of their educational preparation in both undergraduate and graduate programs. Working in clinics, providing education and care to children and families, or serving as medical personnel for missionary teams are just some of the opportunities available to the pediatric generalist and advanced practice nurse. Through the International Council of Nursing (ICN), pediatric nurses can engage in or support larger global issues, such as quality nursing care for all, sound global health policies, the advancement of nursing knowledge, and the presence worldwide of a respected nursing profession and a competent and satisfied nursing workforce. While advances have been made in recent years in the fulfillment of children's rights to survival, health, and education, these gains are in danger of reversal in some parts of the world (Plotnick, 2007). On a global level, the predominant current risks to children are those stemming from poverty, environmental hazards, armed conflict, infectious diseases, and gender inequality.

Complementary Therapies

Increasingly, Americans are turning toward the use of complementary and alternative medicine (CAM) for themselves and their children. CAM is defined as a group of diverse medical and healthcare systems, practices, and products that are not presently considered as part of conventional medicine (National Center for Complementary and Alternative Medicine [NCCAM], 2007). This integrative approach combines conventional treatments with those for which there is high-quality evidence of safety and effectiveness. Examples of complementary and alternative therapies include mind–body techniques (meditation; prayer; creative expression through art, music, or dance), dietary supplements, herbal products, and manipulative or body-based practices such as massage, therapeutic touch, healing touch, Reiki, and magnetic field therapy (NCCAM, 2007). During the 1990s, the utilization of CAM increased from 11% in the early 1990s to 20% by the end of the decade (Ottolini et al., 1999). The use of these therapies for children with chronic illness or fatal conditions or diagnoses is estimated to range from 30–70% depending on patient age and access to service (Breuner, Barry, & Kemper 1998).

CAM is often used in conjunction with other diagnostic, treatment, or prevention strategies. Families who have had a negative experience with conventional medicine may choose alternative or complementary therapies, particularly for children with chronic illnesses. It is important for the pediatric healthcare provider to know what therapies patients and families are using, have a basic working knowledge of such treatments and providers, and be able to talk with families regarding the use of CAM therapies for their children. Also, it is important to assess whether the family has employed cultural practices, ethnic routines, or religious rituals that might include the use of herbs, medicines, or the wearing of certain charms.

Education

Education guidelines for the generalist level of pediatric nursing have been outlined in the *Standards and Guidelines for Pre-licensure and Professional Education for the Nursing Care of Children and Their Families* (Woodring & Pridham, 1998). This document was published with the intent of providing a new vision of education to prepare pre-licensure students and new graduates for the complex care of children and their families. The standards contain 11 concepts in three domains of knowledge and skills that are to be included in every educational program preparing nurses. The document does not produce the curriculum that should be provided within one specific course or set of courses about child health care. Rather, the standards state the goals, process criteria, and outcome criteria for the 11 concepts that can be integrated into all content areas and clinical settings where the needs of children and their families should be discussed. As a collaborator in developing this document, SPN strongly believes that the document serves as a guiding force to direct nursing education for the care of children in our complex society. Pediatric nurses, in collaboration with nursing faculty, help to provide key learning and clinical experiences for students.

Pre-licensure education for the generalist nurse may occur in a variety of programs including baccalaureate and graduate entry programs, associate degree programs, or perhaps a hospital diploma program. In 1986, the AACN published *The Essentials of Baccalaureate Education for Professional Nursing Practice,* a landmark set of core educational standards for the professional nurse. This document was updated in 1998 and is currently undergoing another revision to provide direction for the education of professional nurses in the twenty-first century. *Essentials* defines the professional nurse as "that individual prepared with a minimum of a baccalaureate in nursing but is also inclusive of one who *enters* professional practice with a master's degree in nursing or a nursing doctorate" (AACN, 1998, p. 2).

Educational content regarding genomics and genetics has also been incorporated into nursing curricula. *Essential Nursing Competencies and Curricula Guidelines for Genetics and Genomics*, written by the Consensus Panel on Genetic/Genomic Competencies (2006), outlines the role of the nurse in applying and integrating genetic and genomic knowledge in the processes of screening, assessment, referral, and provision of education, care, and support. This document has been endorsed by numerous nursing organizations including the AAN, ANA, the National League for Nursing, NAPNAP, the National Association of Neonatal Nurses, the National Organization of Nurse Practitioner Faculty (NONPF) and SPN.

Post-baccalaureate education for the advanced practice pediatric nurse is required at the master's or doctoral level. In 1996, the AACN published *The Essentials of Master's Education for Advanced Practice Nursing.* This document outlines a generic core curriculum content for all advanced practice nursing students which includes research, policy, organization and financing of health care, ethics, professional role development, theoretical foundations of nursing practice, human diversity and social issues, and health promotion and disease prevention. A specialty core curriculum for APRNs who provide direct clinical care includes advanced health and physical assessment, advanced pathophysiology, and advanced pharmacology, in additional to clinical experiences.

The National Association of Clinical Nurse Specialists (NACNS) developed a *Statement on CNS Practice and Education* that provides a framework for a first level assessment of core CNS competencies regardless of specialty (NACNS, 2004). Similarly, NONPF (2006b) has developed curriculum guidelines for nurse practitioners, incorporating the full scope of advanced practice nursing. These guidelines and standards apply to graduate education and emphasize direct care across settings. The education of the advanced practice pediatric nurse includes specialty content in advanced health and physical assessment of the child, advanced physiology and pathophysiology, pediatric pharmacology, advanced child and family development, family theory, promotion and mainte-nance of optimal health for children and families, and management of acute and chronic conditions in children.

Clinical practicum experiences for both CNSs and PNPs in a variety of settings are a vital part of the advanced practice curriculum. Clinical experience builds on course work and is designed to enable graduates to collect health data, establish a diagnosis, identify expected outcomes individualized to the child and family, plan and prescribe care, imple-ment interventions, and evaluate the child's and family's progress to-ward attainment of outcomes. In clinical settings, students are expected to provide high-level nursing care based on current clinical evidence and guidelines and which incorporates technical skill, critical thinking, leadership, theoretical knowledge, and clinical scholarship. Academic faculty responsible for the overall implementation of advanced practice programs are ideally prepared at the doctoral level and are actively en-gaged in practice settings with children and families as clinicians, edu-cators, or researchers. Preceptors actively collaborate with educators and students to guide clinical education. Preceptors are nurses who have demonstrated outstanding clinical expertise in a field related to pedi-atric advanced practice. In some academic institutions, preceptors may qualify for courtesy or clinical faculty appointments.

In the past decade, nurse leaders and educators examined the educational programs that prepare advanced practice nurses and reviewed reports and projections for the future healthcare needs of the twenty-first century. It was evident that the educational preparation and provision of services by advanced practice nurses coupled with the com-plexity of healthcare in the United States demanded a transformation. The recommendation was made by the AACN that the future education of advanced practice nurses (clinical nurse specialist and nurse practitioner) would occur at the doctoral level as a Doctor of Nursing Practice (DNP). ANCC recommends that this shift to doctoral preparation should occur by 2015. Additionally, many nurses have and will continue to obtain doc-torate degrees in nursing science and education. These nurses are pre-pared for a wide range of practice environments and responsibilities, including advanced roles in academia, education, and research.

In preparing for this transition in education, the AACN charged a committee to develop *The Essentials of Doctoral Education for Advanced Nursing Practice* (AACN, 2006). This document incorporates and expands on the *Master's Essentials*, currently used to guide advance practice education, to ensure the necessary academic and clinical rigor required for doctoral level education. The eight essentials for doctoral education include:

    I. Scientific underpinnings for practice

    II. Organizational and systems leadership for quality improvement and systems thinking

    III. Clinical scholarship and analytical methods for evidence-based practice

    IV. Information systems and technology, and patient care technology, for the improvement and transformation of health care

    V. Healthcare policy for advocacy in health care

    VI. Interprofessional collaboration for improving patient and population health outcomes

    VII. Clinical prevention and population health for improving the nation's health

    VIII. Advanced nursing practice

Additional work has been done to guide faculty in developing curricula and to set accreditation standards for programs. Advance practice nursing education will now align with audiology, medicine, pharmacy, and physical therapy in preparing practitioners with a terminal doctoral-level practice degree.

Certification

Certification is a process by which an independent, non-governmental agency recognizes an individual nurse's qualifications and knowledge for specialty nursing practice. All pediatric nurses should obtain certification. The nurse achieves specialty certification credentials through the completion of specialized education, experience in specialty nursing practice, and the successful completion of a qualifying examination. Continued certification is accomplished through a variety of mechanisms including re-examination, continuing education, self-assessment, and ongoing clinical practice. Through this process, the agency or professional organization acknowledges for the individual and to the

T A B L E 3 Pediatric Nursing Certification Opportunities

Certifying Organization	Certification Available
American Nurses Credentialing Center (ANCC)	Child/Adolescent Psychiatric and Mental Health Clinical Nurse Specialist, Pediatric Clinical Nurse Specialist, Pediatric Nurse, Pediatric Nurse Practitioner, School Nurse Practitioner*
American Association of Critical Care Nurses: AACCN Certification Corporation	Critical Care Registered Nurse – Pediatric (CCRN-P) Critical Care Registered Nurse – Neonatal (CCRN-N)
Corporation of Pediatric Oncology Nurses (CPON)	Certified Pediatric Oncology Nurse (CPON)
National Board for Certification of School Nurses (NBCSN)	National Certified School Nurse (NCSN)
National Certification Corporation (NCC)	Low-Risk Neonatal Nurse (RNC) Neonatal Intensive Care Nurse (RNC) Neonatal Nurse Practitioner (NNP)
Pediatric Nursing Certification Board (PNCB)	Certified Pediatric Nurse Practitioner – Primary Care (CPNP-PC) Certified Pediatric Nurse Practitioner – Acute Care (CPNP-AC) Certified Pediatric Nurse (CPN)

* Certification is no longer offered

general public that the nurse has mastered a body of knowledge for a particular specialty. Certification is evolving with multiple opportunities for certification available (see Table 3). The nurse should be informed about which certification option is appropriate for him or her.

Regulation

Professional certification is required to practice as a nurse practitioner in most states (Pearson, 2007). State jurisdictions have regulatory and legal oversight of practice for the RN and APRN. There is considerable variability among states in the implementation of this oversight, and APRN statutes vary widely from title protection to a more specific de-lineation of APRN practice. The autonomy of practice ranges from private practice with referral options to practicing under the supervision of a physician. The ANA supports one scope of nursing practice, one licensure for registered nurses, and minimal statutory language about advanced practice. The ANA also proposes that state constituent member associations promote specific designations of APRN roles in rules and regulations instead of law to avoid attaching statutory language to the roles. Additionally, the profession should develop consistent standards of regulation through certification, peer review, and continuing education to self-regulate the role so that the profession retains the responsibility and accountability for regulating practice.

Professional Issues and Trends

Within the broad context of rising healthcare costs, the increasing number of uninsured children and families in the United States, and the consequent disparities in the delivery of health care to those in need, the current professional issues and trends for pediatric nurses are as varied as the settings in which they practice. In acute care and inpatient settings, children with complex diseases are surviving longer, thereby creating new adolescent and young adult populations still needing follow-up care by pediatric healthcare providers in pediatric inpatient units. Thus, creating the need for ongoing education in the areas of adult medicine. Also, many pediatric providers work with chronically ill adolescents in a variety of settings during their transition to adulthood.

With the development of new vaccines, the percentage of pediatric inpatient admissions for infectious disease has declined. As noted above, more parents are turning towards the use of CAM therapies as an adjunct to conventional medical treatments in treating their children. For advanced practice pediatric nurses in primary and specialty care settings, additional clinical challenges include providing care for children who present with chronic health problems that stem from complications of overweight and obesity, asthma and allergic conditions, and behavioral and mental health concerns.

More children's hospitals are seeking Magnet Status from the American Nurses Credentialing Center (ANCC), which identifies institutions as meeting set standards for the provision of excellent nursing care. Because of this pursuit, pediatric nurses in both general and advanced practice are seeking certification and advanced educational degrees.

Professionally, nurses continue to address issues of entry into practice, the autonomy of advanced practice, multiple certification pathways, and the various educational credentials appropriate for certification. Overall, efforts must be made to narrow the gap between the abilities of healthcare providers and the activities which governmental regulation prevents them from performing (Safriet 2002). Nurses must continue to demonstrate to the payers of health care and to the public the value of an interdisciplinary system which provides efficient, quality health care.

Ethical Issues in Pediatric Care

Pediatric care is delivered in an environment of specialized knowledge and skill under circumstances in which opportunities for ethical deliberation and reflection may be less than ideal. Parents and families are emotionally stressed, and in some instances they themselves may be patients. Staffing and other organizational issues may introduce additional stress on the care team apart from the dynamics of a particular case. These examples only emphasize the importance of viewing the pediatric care unit as a moral community in which ethical reflection, discussion, and action are as much a part of a care plan as diagnosis and treatment. Viewing ethics in this context also allows for an understanding of ethical issues that is both deep and broad, encompassing ethical distress that may occur within one's self, among members of the care team, and between the care team and families.

The values of advocacy, respect for persons, and justice are among those that have been identified by nurses as societal values with particular relevance to the profession of nursing. Thus, as a member of the profession, each individual nurse has accepted the ethical obligations of the role in addition to the individual capacity to make moral choices as human beings. While this provides a rich legacy, it can also be a source of ethical uncertainty or conflict when the care plan for a particular patient or institutional rules require some sacrifice of one's individual moral code in carrying out professional responsibilities. In some cases, a healthy professional distance allows us to carry out decisions that are ethically permissible even though they are not the choices we would make for our own children.

Occasionally, however, a case presents itself in which taking this course is not easily reconciled. Prolonged life-supporting therapy that is insisted on by parents and allowed by physicians may in some cases compromise both a nurse's professional identity and personal moral agency. How such situations are handled is as ethically important as the course of action one chooses to take.

How pediatric nurses understand what an ethical dilemma is can influence their ability to identify ethical issues, discuss them with colleagues, and take action to resolve or ameliorate ethical conflict. Differences within the healthcare team may be enriched or impeded by different cultural and religious backgrounds and by hierarchical and power differentials that are often unspoken but powerful influences in how a unit functions. Understanding the unit as a moral community includes not only how we treat patients, but also how nurses treat each other. All members of the healthcare team must have a realistic understanding of ethics as an everyday concern rather than an issue of crisis management, so that an environment is created in which high standards are the rule rather than the exception, providing support for a community characterized by mutual respect and willingness to take responsibility for lapses and improvements.

Although there is a tendency to put difficult cases behind oneself as quickly as possible and move on, ethical growth requires that nurses reflect on our practice so that one can identify and reinforce what one does well and learn from one's inexperience and mistakes. Nursing codes of ethics provide principles based on important moral values that shape the nurse's professional identity (ANA, 2001) and provide the nurse the foundation to apply the principles in his or her work setting.

Advocacy in Pediatric Care

Every pediatric nurse is a child advocate. Advocacy can occur in the hospital setting, ambulatory care setting, educational setting, committee meetings, agency discussions, parent meetings, and public settings, sometimes on a daily basis. Advocacy means providing a voice for those who are not heard, ensuring that important issues are addressed (Sullivan 2004). Pediatric nurses hold many qualities that are needed for advocating: strong communication skills, the ability to negotiate, awareness of patient needs, perseverance, leadership and people skills, and the ability to both multitask and think innovatively "outside the workplace". The specialized knowledge that pediatric nurses possess, combined with their holistic approach and their understanding of the context of child health, can assist in the creation, implementation, and evaluation of policies at all levels. Pediatric nurses can be involved in advocacy by finding their passion related to their work, community, or personal interests which can all lead to avenues of advocacy. Being involved in committees in the workplace, committees for professional associations, and involvement in community activities are examples of advocacy opportunities.

Pediatric nurses understand both the pediatric patient and family needs, which places them in a prime position to advocate for those identified needs. Because of their expertise, the pediatric nurse can see the effects of policy decisions on the health and well-being of the patient and family. Professional values of possessing an ethical framework, abiding by the code of ethics for nurses (ANA, 2001), and acknowledging the mission and goals of professional organizations can guide the nurse in advocacy efforts. Advocacy success has been demonstrated in areas surrounding the development of safe playgrounds, choking prevention, ensuring healthier school lunch programs, and assuring funding and services in state children's health insurance programs (SCHIP).

Continued Commitment to the Profession

Pediatric healthcare professionals are committed to:

- demonstrating excellent nursing practice consistent with professional nursing standards, specialty nursing standards, and state boards of registered nursing regulations for generalist and advanced practice nurses;
- supporting education and role development of novice practitioners by serving as preceptors, role models, and mentors;
- advancing the profession through enhancing public awareness and community activities;
- maintaining active membership in professional organizations;
- working to influence policy-making bodies to improve access to quality health care;
- using an ethical framework to evaluate issues regarding care; and

- demonstrating practice consistent with ethical and legal standards in compliance with state and federal regulations.

Furthermore, pediatric nurses are committed to working together to address the common issues that affect pediatric nurses who practice in diverse roles and settings and who may belong to varied professional pediatric organizations. In so doing, they are able to effectively merge their knowledge, insights, resources, and goals for the future, and thereby improve the health care of the children and families to whom they are ultimately accountable.

STANDARDS OF PEDIATRIC NURSING PRACTICE
STANDARDS OF PRACTICE

STANDARD 1. ASSESSMENT
The pediatric nurse collects comprehensive data pertinent to the patient's health or the situation.

Measurement Criteria:

The Pediatric Nurse:

- Collects data in a systematic and ongoing process that conveys respect for the child and family.

- Involves the child, family, other individuals important to the family, and other healthcare providers, as appropriate, in holistic data collection.

- Utilizes the preferred language of the family through a culturally sensitive process, and seeks a qualified interpreter if necessary.

- Assesses the child's and family's environment.

- Prioritizes data collection activities based on the child's immediate condition, situation, and anticipated needs.

- Uses appropriate evidence-based assessment techniques specific for the child's age in collecting pertinent data.

  - Physical assessment may include but not be limited to:

    - Height, weight (current and pre-illness), body mass index (BMI)

    - Vital signs including pain assessment

    - Hearing and vision screening

    - Tanner staging of pubertal development

    - Nutritional status

    - Physical examination

    - Head circumference (age-appropriate)

Continued ▶

- Behavioral assessment may include but not be limited to:
  - Tolerance of the physical examination or procedures
  - Affect and activity
  - Interactions with adults and peers
  - Behavioral differences across settings (home, school, clinic, hospital)
- Developmental assessment may include but not be limited to:
  - Personal characteristics and social skills
  - Language
  - Fine motor and adaptive
  - Gross motor
  - Cognitive
  - Emotional and mental health
  - Temperament
  - Moral development
- Family assessment may include:
  - Determining who the child lives with
  - Familial strengths
  - Cultural background
  - Ethnic background
  - Socioeconomic background
  - Mental health issues
  - Religious or spiritual background
  - Coping strategies
  - Learning style
  - Injury prevention and safety practices
  - Preferences of family for receiving information and support
  - Ways the family can partner in providing the child's health care

- Health history may include but not be limited to:
  - Birth history (age-appropriate)
  - Growth and development milestones
  - Past medical illness or surgeries
  - Medications and allergies
  - Family history, including genetic history and congenital abnormalities
  - Mental or emotional disabilities, metabolic problems, and chronic health problems
  - Accidents or injuries
  - Educational needs related to maximizing the child's health
  - Behavioral patterns and individual strengths
  - Communicable or childhood diseases
  - Exposure to hazardous agents
  - Dietary habits and intake history
  - Growth parameters as compared with normal for age
  - Significant trends in weight gain or loss
  - Immunization status
  - Sexual history (age-appropriate)
  - Substance abuse history (age-appropriate)
  - Engagement in high-risk activities (smoking, drugs or alcohol, body piercing or tattoos, sexual activity, performance-enhancing drugs)
  - Experience with pain and pain management techniques
  - School history (age-appropriate)
  - Elimination patterns
  - Sleep patterns and sleep aids
  - Information that family member sees as significant

Continued ▶

- Family observations of the child
- Strengths of the child and family
- Any significant stressors; comforting and coping strategies
- Relationships with the family, including potential for abuse
- Socioeconomic, cultural, spiritual, and environmental factors
- Peer relationships
- Travel history

- Uses analytical models and problem-solving tools to systematically collect data.
- Synthesizes available data, information, and knowledge relevant to the situation to identify patterns and variances.
- Documents relevant data in a retrievable form.
- Bases assessment techniques on research and knowledge, using clinical judgment to ensure that relevant and necessary data are collected.

Additional Measurement Criteria for the Advanced Practice Pediatric Nurse:

The Advanced Practice Pediatric Nurse:

- Initiates and interprets age-appropriate and condition-specific laboratory tests and diagnostic procedures.

STANDARD 2. DIAGNOSIS
The pediatric nurse analyzes the assessment data to determine the diagnoses or healthcare issues.

Measurement Criteria:

The Pediatric Nurse:

- Derives the diagnoses or issues based on assessment data.

- Derives diagnoses that are developmentally appropriate and specific to areas of growth and development, age, cultural sensitivity, and family dynamics.

- Validates the prioritized diagnoses or issues with the child, family, significant others, and other healthcare providers when possible and appropriate.

- Documents diagnoses or issues in a manner that facilitates the determination of the expected outcomes and plan of care.

Additional Measurement Criteria for the Advanced Practice Pediatric Nurse:

The Advanced Practice Pediatric Nurse:

- Systematically compares and contrasts clinical findings with normal and abnormal variations and developmental events in formulating a differential diagnosis.

- Determines diagnoses related to disease and injury prevention and health promotion, restoration, and maintenance.

- Utilizes complex data and information obtained during interview, examination, and diagnostic procedures in identifying diagnoses.

- Revises diagnoses as appropriate to the ongoing evaluation.

- Conforms diagnosis to an accepted classification system (as may be defined by the healthcare setting).

- Assists staff in developing and maintaining competency in the diagnostic process.

STANDARD 3. OUTCOMES IDENTIFICATION
The pediatric nurse identifies expected outcomes for a plan of care individualized to the child, family, and the situation.

Measurement Criteria:

The Pediatric Nurse:

- Involves the child (when age appropriate), family, and other health-care providers in formulating expected outcomes when possible and appropriate.

- Derives outcomes that are developmentally appropriate, age-specific, family centered, and culturally sensitive.

- Derives outcomes that are realistic in relation to the child's and family's potential capabilities and available resources.

- Considers associated risks, benefits, costs, current scientific evidence, and clinical expertise when formulating expected outcomes.

- Defines expected outcomes in terms of the child, the child's values, ethical considerations, environment or situation with consideration of risks, benefits and costs, and current scientific evidence.

- Includes a time estimate for attainment of expected outcomes, and prioritizes as appropriate.

- Develops expected outcomes that provide direction for continuity of care.

- Identifies expected outcomes that incorporate scientific evidence and are achievable through implementation of evidence-based practices.

- Modifies expected outcomes based on changes in the status of the child or evaluation of the situation.

- Documents expected outcomes as measurable goals.

Additional Measurement Criteria for the Advanced Practice Pediatric Nurse:

The Advanced Practice Pediatric Nurse:

- Identifies expected outcomes with consideration of the associated risks, benefits, and costs for the child and family.

- Identifies expected outcomes that incorporate cost and clinical effectiveness, the child's and family's satisfaction, and continuity and consistency among providers.

- Supports the use of clinical guidelines linked to positive outcomes for the child.

STANDARD 4. PLANNING
The pediatric nurse develops a plan of care that prescribes strategies and alternatives to attain expected outcomes.

Measurement Criteria:

The Pediatric Nurse:

- Develops an individualized plan of care considering the child's characteristics or the situation (including age, growth, developmental, cultural, and environmental factors).

- Develops the plan of care in conjunction with the child (when developmentally able), family, and others, as appropriate.

- Formulates a plan of care that is family centered and reflects current pediatric nursing practice, and takes into consideration the family's cultural needs, ability to read and write, level of health literacy, and capacity for understanding complex healthcare processes.

- Includes strategies within the plan of care that address each of the identified diagnoses or issues, which may include strategies for promotion and restoration of health and prevention of illness, injury, and disease.

- Provides for continuity within the plan of care.

- Provides for confidentiality when necessary.

- Incorporates an implementation pathway or timeline within the plan of care that is dynamic, flexible, and reassessed as needed.

- Re-evaluates the plan of care with the child, family, and others as appropriate.

- Utilizes the plan of care to provide direction to other members of the healthcare team.

- Defines the plan of care to reflect current statutes, rules and regulations, and standards.

- Integrates current trends and research affecting care in the planning process.

- Considers the economic impact of the plan of care.

- Uses standardized language or recognized terminology to document the plan of care.

- Documents the plan of care.

Additional Measurement Criteria for the Advanced Practice Pediatric Nurse:

The Advanced Practice Pediatric Nurse:

- Identifies assessment, diagnostic strategies, and therapeutic interventions within the plan of care that reflect current pediatric health-care practice, including data, research, literature, and expert clinical knowledge.

- Devises a comprehensive plan of care that reflects the responsibilities of the advanced practice nurse, the child, and the family and may include delegation of responsibilities and consultation to assist others in implementing the plan of care.

- Participates in the design and development of multidisciplinary and interdisciplinary processes to address the situation or issue.

- Formulates the comprehensive plan of care that includes educational interventions related to the child's health status, conventional and alternative therapies, self-care activities, and appropriate referrals and coordination of comprehensive services to ensure continuity of care.

- Documents the comprehensive plan of care in a manner that allows access by the child, the family, and healthcare providers as appropriate, and provides direction for the family and the healthcare team as they focus on attaining expected outcomes.

- Selects or designs strategies to meet the multifaceted needs of the complex pediatric patient.

- Includes the synthesis of the child's and family's values and beliefs regarding nursing and medical therapies within the plan of care.

- Contributes to the development and continuous improvement of organizational systems that support the plan of care process.

- Supports the integration of clinical, human, and financial resources to enhance and complete the decision-making processes.

STANDARD 5. IMPLEMENTATION
The pediatric nurse implements the identified plan of care.

Measurement Criteria:

The Pediatric Nurse:

- Performs interventions that are consistent with the established plan of care and are family centered, developmentally appropriate, age specific, and culturally sensitive.

- Encourages the child of accountable age and ability to assume responsibility related to his or her care.

- Provides to the child or the caregiver education that includes health promotion, anticipatory guidance, information about injury and disease prevention, and home care management as appropriate for the child's developmental level.

- Counsels the child and family in resolving issues or making determinations of what the next appropriate steps might be. Implements the plan of care in a safe, cost-effective, and timely manner.

- Documents implementation and any modifications, including changes or omissions, of the identified plan of care.

- Utilizes evidence-based interventions and treatments specific to the diagnosis or problem.

- Utilizes community resources and systems to implement the plan of care, and coordinates access to the appropriate resources.

- Collaborates with nursing colleagues and others to implement the plan of care.

Additional Measurement Criteria for the Advanced Practice Pediatric Nurse:

The Advanced Practice Pediatric Nurse:

- Facilitates utilization of systems and community resources to implement the plan of care.

- Supports collaboration with nursing colleagues and other disciplines to implement the plan of care.

- Incorporates new knowledge and strategies to initiate change in nursing care practices if desired outcomes are not achieved.

- Implements interventions and treatments that are based on current clinical evidence and theory.

- Performs interventions and treatments for which the nurse has received appropriate training and has demonstrated competency in the skill or procedure being performed.

- Implements the plan of care using principles and concepts of project or systems management.

- Fosters organizational systems that support implementation of the plan of care.

STANDARD 5A: COORDINATION OF CARE AND CASE MANAGEMENT
The pediatric nurse coordinates care delivery.

Measurement Criteria:

The Pediatric Nurse:

- Coordinates implementation of the plan of care.

- Documents the coordination of the care.

- Communicates with all healthcare providers involved in the child's care.

Additional Measurement Criteria for the Advanced Practice Pediatric Nurse:

The Advanced Practice Pediatric Nurse:

- Provides leadership in the coordination of multidisciplinary health care for integrated delivery of pediatric care services.

- Delegates appropriate monitoring, assessments, and interventions according to the condition of the child and the relative skill and scope of practice of the caregiver.

- Provides case management and clinical coordination of care using sophisticated data synthesis with consideration of the child's and family's complex needs and desired outcomes.

- Coordinates system and community resources to achieve optimal quality of care, delivered in a cost-effective manner within an interdisciplinary team approach.

- Negotiates health-related services and additional specialized care with the child, the family, appropriate systems, agencies, and providers across continuums of care.

STANDARD 5B: HEALTH TEACHING AND HEALTH PROMOTION, RESTORATION AND MAINTENANCE

The pediatric nurse employs strategies to promote health and a safe environment.

Measurement Criteria:

The Pediatric Nurse:

- Provides health teaching that addresses such topics as healthy lifestyles, risk-reducing behaviors, developmental needs, activities of daily living, and preventive self-care and is based on current scientific knowledge, research, epidemiological principles, and the family's health beliefs and practices.

- Uses health promotion and health teaching methods appropriate to the situation and to the child's and family's developmental levels, learning needs, readiness, ability to learn, language preference, and culture.

- Provides information on the risks and benefits of healthcare practices.

- Seeks opportunities for feedback and evaluation of the effectiveness of the strategies used.

- Designs health information and pediatric education appropriate to the child's culture, age, developmental and cognitive levels, and readiness and ability to learn.

- Evaluates health information resources, such as the Internet, within the area of practice for accuracy, readability, and comprehensibility to help the child and the family access quality health information.

Additional Measurement Criteria for the Advanced Practice Pediatric Nurse:

The Advanced Practice Pediatric Nurse:

- Employs diverse and complex strategies, interventions, and teaching with the child and the family to promote, maintain, restore, and improve health, and to prevent illness and injury.

Continued ▶

- Synthesizes empirical evidence on risk behaviors, learning theories, behavioral change theories, motivational theories, epidemiology, and other related theories and frameworks when designing health information and pediatric education.

- Bases anticipatory guidance and teaching on current scientific knowledge, research, epidemiological principles, and the family's health beliefs and practices.

- Provides the child (if age appropriate) and the family information regarding the interventions including potential benefits, risks, complications, and alternatives.

STANDARD 5c: CONSULTATION

The pediatric nurse provides consultation to healthcare providers and others to influence the identified plan of care for children, to enhance the abilities of others to provide health care, and to effect change in the healthcare system.

Measurement Criteria:

The Pediatric Nurse:

- Synthesizes data, information, theoretical frameworks, and evidence when providing consultation.

- Facilitates the effectiveness of a consultation by involving the stakeholders in the decision-making process.

- Communicates consultation recommendations that influence the identified plan of care, facilitate understanding by involved stakeholders, enhance the work of others, and effect change.

Additional Measurement Criteria for the Advanced Practice Pediatric Nurse:

The Advanced Practice Pediatric Nurse:

- Bases consultative activities on theoretical frameworks, including those that focus on family systems and family-centered care, and on evidence for best practice.

- Bases consultation on mutual respect among the child, the family, and other primary caregivers.

- Initiates consultation through mutual identification of the needs for intervention and problem identification

- Initiates appropriate consultation to implement the interdisciplinary plan of care for the child with consideration given to the child's unique developmental needs and abilities and the family's level of adaptation and ability to cope with the child's health concerns.

- Communicates consultation recommendations in terms that facilitate change.

- Supports the child and the family in their decision-making regarding the implementation of the plan of care.

STANDARD 5D: PRESCRIPTIVE AUTHORITY AND TREATMENT
The advanced practice pediatric nurse utilizes prescriptive authority, procedures, referrals, treatments, and therapies in providing care.

Measurement Criteria for the Advanced Practice Pediatric Nurse:

The Advanced Practice Pediatric Nurse:

- Prescribes evidence-based treatments, therapies, and procedures considering the child's comprehensive healthcare needs and based on current pediatric knowledge, research, and practice.

- Prescribes appropriate non-pharmacological interventions, including complementary and alternative therapies.

- Performs procedures as needed in the delivery of comprehensive care to the child.

- Prescribes pharmacologic agents based on current knowledge of pharmacological and physiological principles that are both universal and unique to the care of children at each stage in their development.

- Prescribes specific pharmacological agents and treatments based on clinical indicators, the child's status and needs, and the results of diagnostic and laboratory tests.

- Provides the child (if age appropriate) and family with information about diagnostic and laboratory results, as well as effects and potential adverse effects of proposed prescriptive therapies.

- Evaluates therapeutic and potential adverse effects of pharmacological and non-pharmacological treatments.

- Provides information to the family regarding agents the child should refrain from taking because of the potential adverse effects on the child.

- Provides the child (if age appropriate) and family with information about costs, alternative treatments, and procedures, as appropriate.

- Monitors current issues related to pharmacological agents, including off-label use and pediatric safe dosage for medications indicated for adults.

STANDARD 5E: REFERRAL

The advanced practice pediatric nurse identifies the need for additional care and makes referrals as indicated.

Measurement Criteria:

The Advanced Practice Pediatric Nurse:

- Discusses referrals with the child (if age appropriate) and family.

- Makes referrals to other healthcare providers and community service agencies as appropriate to the needs of the child with consideration of benefits and costs.

- Ensures continuity of care throughout the healthcare referral process by implementing recommendations from referral sources.

- Identifies and coordinates access to appropriate community resources.

STANDARD 6. EVALUATION
The pediatric nurse evaluates progress towards attainment of outcomes.

Measurement Criteria:

The Pediatric Nurse:

- Conducts a systematic, ongoing, and criterion-based evaluation of the outcomes in relation to the structures and processes prescribed by the plan of care and the indicated timeline.

- Includes the child, family, and other healthcare providers involved in the care or situation in the evaluation process.

- Evaluates the effectiveness of the plan of care strategies in relation to the child's responses and the attainment of the expected outcomes.

- Documents the results of the evaluation.

- Uses ongoing assessment data to revise the diagnoses, outcomes, the plan of care, and the implementation as needed.

- Documents revisions in diagnoses, outcomes, and the plan of care.

- Documents the child's and the family's readiness for and responses to interventions.

- Disseminates evaluation results to the child (if age appropriate), the family, and others involved in the care or situation, as appropriate.

Additional Measurement Criteria for the Advanced Practice Pediatric Nurse:

The Advanced Practice Pediatric Nurse:

- Evaluates the accuracy of the diagnosis and effectiveness of the interventions in relationship to the child's attainment of expected outcomes.

- Bases the evaluation process on advanced knowledge, practice, and research about child health care.

- Utilizes results of evaluation analyses to revise or resolve the diagnoses, expected outcomes, and plan of care.

- Synthesizes the results of the evaluation analyses to determine the impact of the plan of care on the affected child, family, groups, communities, institutions, networks, and organizations

- Utilizes the results of the evaluation analyses to make or recommend process or structural changes including policy, procedure, or protocol documentation as appropriate.

STANDARDS OF PROFESSIONAL PERFORMANCE

STANDARD 7. QUALITY OF PRACTICE
The pediatric nurse systematically enhances the quality and effectiveness of nursing practice.

Measurement Criteria:

The Pediatric Nurse:

- Demonstrates quality by documenting the application of the nursing process and evidence-based practice in a responsible, accountable, and ethical manner.

- Uses the results of quality improvement activities to initiate changes in pediatric nursing practice and in the healthcare delivery system, and communicates results to others who may benefit.

- Uses creativity and innovation in pediatric nursing practice to improve care delivery to children and families.

- Incorporates new knowledge to initiate changes in nursing practice if desired outcomes are not achieved.

- Participates in quality improvement activities. Such activities may include:

  - Identifying aspects of practice important for quality monitoring.

  - Using indicators developed to monitor quality and effectiveness of nursing practice.

  - Collecting data to monitor quality and effectiveness of nursing practice.

  - Analyzing quality data to identify opportunities for improving nursing practice.

  - Formulating recommendations to improve nursing practice or outcomes.

  - Developing, implementing, and evaluating activities, policies, procedures, and guidelines to improve the quality of practice.

Continued ▶

- Participating on interdisciplinary teams to improve the care delivery process and patient outcomes.

- Participating in efforts to minimize costs and unnecessary duplication.

- Analyzing factors related to safety, satisfaction, effectiveness, and cost–benefit options.

- Analyzing organizational systems for barriers.

- Implementing processes to remove or decrease barriers within organizational systems.

Additional Measurement Criteria for the Advanced Practice Pediatric Nurse:

The Advanced Practice Pediatric Nurse:

- Designs quality improvement initiatives.

- Implements initiatives to evaluate the need for change.

- Evaluates the practice environment and quality of nursing care rendered in relation to existing evidence, identifying opportunities for the generation and translation of research findings.

- Obtains and maintains professional certification in advanced practice pediatric nursing.

- Provides leadership in establishing and monitoring standards of practice to improve care of children and their families in collaboration with other healthcare team members.

- Participates in efforts to minimize costs and unnecessary duplication of tests and diagnostic services, and facilitates the timely provision of services for the child and the family.

- Analyzes factors related to safety, satisfaction, effectiveness, and cost–benefit options with the child, family, and other healthcare providers as appropriate.

- Identifies and works to remove barriers in organizational systems that may hinder the quality of pediatric nursing care.

STANDARD 8. PROFESSIONAL PRACTICE EVALUATION

The pediatric nurse evaluates one's own nursing practice in relation to professional practice standards and guidelines, relevant statutes, rules, and regulations.

Measurement Criteria:

The Pediatric Nurse:

- Evaluates one's own cultural and ethnic sensitivity when providing care.

- Engages in self-evaluation of practice on a regular basis, identifying areas of strength as well as areas in which professional development would be beneficial.

- Obtains informal feedback regarding one's own practice from the child and family, peers, professional colleagues, and others.

- Participates in systematic peer review as appropriate.

- Takes action to achieve goals identified during the evaluation process.

- Provides rationale for practice beliefs, decisions, and actions as part of the informal and formal evaluation processes.

- Applies knowledge of current professional practice standards, guidelines, statutes, rules, and regulations that affect the nursing care of children and families.

- Evaluates performance according to the standards of the profession and the standards specific to pediatric nursing and various regulatory bodies, and takes action to improve practice.

- Analyzes the effectiveness of interventions, the incidence and types of complications, and child outcome data to improve practice.

- Takes action to achieve goals identified during performance appraisal and peer review, resulting in changes in practice and role performance.

- Synthesizes and uses the results of evaluation to make or recommend changes including policy, procedure, or protocol documentation.

Continued ▶

Additional Measurement Criteria for the Advanced Practice Pediatric Nurse:

The Advanced Practice Pediatric Nurse:

- Engages in a formal process seeking feedback regarding one's own practice from the child, family, peers, professional colleagues, and others.

Standard 9. Education
The pediatric nurse attains knowledge and competency that reflects current nursing practice.

Measurement Criteria:

The Pediatric Nurse:

- Participates in ongoing nursing and interdisciplinary educational activities related to clinical knowledge and professional issues.

- Demonstrates a commitment to lifelong learning through self-reflection and inquiry to identify learning needs.

- Seeks experiences that reflect current pediatric nursing practice in order to maintain skills and competence in clinical practice or role performance.

- Acquires culturally competent and clinically sound knowledge and skills appropriate to the health care of children and their families, and to the practice setting, role, or situation.

- Maintains professional records that provide evidence of competency and lifelong learning.

- Seeks experiences as well as formal and independent learning activities to maintain and develop clinical and professional skills and knowledge.

Additional Measurement Criteria for the Advanced Practice Pediatric Nurse:

The Advanced Practice Pediatric Nurse:

- Utilizes current healthcare research findings and other evidence to expand clinical knowledge, enhance role performance, and increase knowledge of professional issues.

- Supports the education and role development of other practitioners by serving as preceptor, role model, and mentor.

STANDARD 10. COLLEGIALITY

The pediatric nurse interacts with and contributes to the professional development of peers and colleagues.

Measurement Criteria:

The Pediatric Nurse:

- Shares knowledge and skills with peers and colleagues as evidenced by such activities as child care conferences or presentations at formal or informal meetings.

- Provides peers with feedback regarding their practice and role performance.

- Interacts with peers and colleagues to enhance one's own professional nursing practice and role performance.

- Maintains compassionate and caring relationships with peers and colleagues.

- Contributes to an environment that is conducive to the clinical education of nursing students and other healthcare professionals.

- Contributes to a supportive and healthy work environment.

Additional Measurement Criteria for the Advanced Practice Pediatric Nurse:

The Advanced Practice Pediatric Nurse:

- Models expert practice to interdisciplinary team members and healthcare consumers.

- Participates on interdisciplinary teams that contribute to role development, advanced pediatric nursing practice, and health care.

- Contributes to an environment that is conducive to clinical education of other healthcare providers, including teaching, mentoring, and precepting.

- Contributes to the professional development of others to improve child health care and to foster the profession's growth.

Standard 11. Collaboration
The pediatric nurse collaborates with the child, family, and others in the conduct of nursing practice.

Measurement Criteria:

The Pediatric Nurse:

- Communicates with child, family, and others regarding health care of the child and the nurse's role in providing that care.

- Collaborates with the interdisciplinary and intradisciplinary health-care teams and family in creating a documented plan of care focusing on outcomes and decisions related to patient care and delivery of services.

- Partners with others to effect change and generate positive outcomes through knowledge of the child or situation.

- Documents referrals, including provision for continuity of care.

- Assists the family in identifying and accessing community resources to support the family in the care of the child as appropriate.

Additional Measurement Criteria for the Advanced Practice Pediatric Nurse:

The Advanced Practice Pediatric Nurse:

- Partners with other disciplines to enhance pediatric health care through interdisciplinary activities, such as education, consultation, development of new management and therapeutic strategies or research.

- Facilitates an interdisciplinary process with other members of the healthcare team.

- Documents plans, communications, management plan changes, and collaborative discussions to improve pediatric health care.

STANDARD 12. ETHICS

The pediatric nurse integrates ethical considerations and processes in all areas of practice.

Measurement Criteria:

The Pediatric Nurse:

- Uses *Code of Ethics for Nurses with Interpretive Statements* (ANA 2001) to guide practice.

- Delivers care in a manner that preserves and protects the child's and family's autonomy, dignity, and rights.

- Delivers care in a nonjudgmental and nondiscriminatory manner that is sensitive to and values diversity.

- Maintains confidentiality within legal and regulatory parameters.

- Enables children and families to participate in ethical decision-making processes.

- Maintains a therapeutic and professional relationship with appropriate professional role boundaries.

- Demonstrates a commitment to practicing self-care, managing stress, and connecting with self and others.

- Facilitates family participation in ethical decision-making.

- Contributes to multidisciplinary teams or committees that address ethical questions, benefits, and outcomes.

- Informs administrators or others of the risks, benefits, and outcomes of programs and decisions that affect healthcare delivery.

- Reports abuse of patients' rights and incompetent, unethical, or illegal practice.

Additional Measurement Criteria for the Advanced Practice Pediatric Nurse:

The Advanced Practice Pediatric Nurse:

- Ensures that the care provided is consistent with the child's and family's needs and values, and with codes of ethical practice.

- Informs the child (as appropriate) and family of the risks, benefits, and outcomes of healthcare regimens.

- Makes decisions and initiates actions on behalf of children and their families in an ethical manner, taking into consideration the values of the child and family.

- Ensures informed consent or age-appropriate assent for procedures, treatment, and research, as appropriate.

- Serves as an advocate for the child and family in developing policies and in providing care to the child and family.

- Contributes to the creation of individual and system responses to resolution of ethical dilemmas.

- Advocates for a process of ongoing ethical inquiry into patient care practices where varying perspectives are acknowledged and validated.

STANDARD 13. RESEARCH, EVIDENCE-BASED PRACTICE, AND CLINICAL SCHOLARSHIP

The pediatric nurse integrates research findings into practice and, where appropriate, participates in the generation of new knowledge.

Measurement Criteria:

The Pediatric Nurse:

- Utilizes the best available evidence, including research findings, to guide practice decisions.

- Protects the rights of all children and families involved in research studies.

- Actively participates in research activities at various levels appropriate to the nurse's level of education, position, and practice environment. Such activities may include:

  - Identifying clinical problems or questions suitable for nursing research.

  - Identifying possible candidates to be enrolled in studies.

  - Participating in data collection.

  - Participating in a formal committee or program.

  - Sharing research activities and findings with peers and others.

  - Conducting research.

  - Critically analyzing and interpreting research for application to practice.

  - Translating research findings in the development of policies, procedures, and standards of practice for the delivery of pediatric health care.

  - Incorporating research as a basis for learning.

Additional Measurement Criteria for the Advanced Practice Pediatric Nurse:

The Advanced Practice Pediatric Nurse:

- Contributes to nursing knowledge by conducting or synthesizing research that discovers, examines, and evaluates knowledge, theories, criteria, and creative approaches to improve healthcare practice.

- Formally and informally disseminates research findings through practice, education, presentations, publications, consultation, and journal clubs.

STANDARD 14. RESOURCE UTILIZATION

The pediatric nurse considers factors related to safety, effectiveness, cost, and impact on practice in planning and delivering patient care.

Measurement Criteria:

The Pediatric Nurse:

- Evaluates factors such as safety, effectiveness, availability, cost and benefits, efficiencies, and impact on practice when choosing practice options that would result in the same expected outcome.

- Assists the child and family in identifying and securing appropriate and available services to address health-related needs.

- Assigns or delegates tasks, based on the needs and condition of the child, potential for harm, stability of the child's condition, complexity of the task, and predictability of the outcome.

- Assists the child and family in becoming informed consumers about the options, costs, risks, and benefits of treatment and care.

- Assists the family in identifying and accessing resources for pediatric patients requiring long-term or rehabilitative care.

Additional Measurement Criteria for the Advanced Practice Pediatric Nurse:

The Advanced Practice Pediatric Nurse:

- Utilizes organizational and community resources to formulate multidisciplinary or interdisciplinary plans of care.

- Develops innovative solutions for child healthcare problems that address effective resource utilization and maintenance of quality.

- Develops evaluation strategies to demonstrate cost effectiveness, cost– benefit, and efficiency factors associated with pediatric nursing practice.

- Develops evaluation methods to measure safety and effectiveness for interventions and outcomes.

- Promotes activities that assist others, as appropriate, in becoming informed about costs, risks, and benefits of care or of the plan of care and solution.

- Initiates ongoing activities to analyze patient care systems in an effort to improve the quality of care provided to children and their families.

- Uses aggregate data, in cooperation with others, to develop or revise systems to avoid duplication of or gaps in service.

- Advocates for the removal of barriers to care and for optimal care for the child and family.

- Develops innovative solutions and applies strategies to obtain appropriate resources for nursing initiatives.

- Secures organizational resources to ensure a work environment conducive to completing the identified plan of care and outcomes.

STANDARD 15. LEADERSHIP
The pediatric nurse provides leadership in the professional practice setting and the profession.

Measurement Criteria:

The Pediatric Nurse:

- Engages in teamwork as a team leader or team member.

- Works to create and maintain healthy work environments in local, regional, national, or international communities.

- Displays the ability to define a clear vision, the associated goals, and a plan of care to implement and measure progress.

- Demonstrates a commitment to continuous, lifelong learning for self and others.

- Teaches others to succeed by mentoring and other strategies.

- Exhibits creativity and flexibility through times of change.

- Demonstrates energy, excitement, and a passion for quality work.

- Willingly accepts and is accountable for errors by self and others, thereby creating a culture in which risk-taking is not only safe, but also expected.

- Inspires loyalty through the valuing of people as the most precious asset in an organization.

- Directs the coordination of care across settings and among caregivers, including oversight of licensed and unlicensed personnel in any assigned or delegated tasks.

- Serves in key roles in the work setting by participating on committees, councils, and administrative teams.

- Promotes advancement of the profession through participation in professional organizations.

Additional Measurement Criteria for the Advanced Practice Pediatric Nurse:

The Advanced Practice Pediatric Nurse:

- Works to influence decision-making bodies to improve child healthcare, health services, and policies.

- Provides direction to enhance the effectiveness of the multi-disciplinary healthcare team.

- Initiates and revises protocols or guidelines to reflect evidence-based practice, accepted changes in care management, or to address emerging problems.

- Promotes communication of information and advancement of the profession through writing, publishing, and presentations for professional or lay audiences.

- Designs innovations to effect change in practice and improve health outcomes.

STANDARD 16. ADVOCACY

The pediatric nurse is an advocate for the pediatric client and family.

Measurement Criteria:

The Pediatric Nurse:

- Advocates for organizational, environmental, and practice changes to ensure that the unique health needs of children are met.

- Assists children and families to adjust to the changing healthcare environment.

- Protects the human and legal rights of the pediatric patient and family.

- Serves as a leader for the purpose of influencing healthcare practice and policy in the care of children, families, and communities.

- Assists the pediatric client and family in decision-making regarding healthcare choices.

- Provides pediatric clients and families with informed choices.

- Advocates for the child, and works with families, social service agencies, and the courts when there is concern about child abuse, neglect, or other forms of family violence.

- Raises public awareness about issues related to the health care of children and families.

- Participates in legislative agendas that improve healthcare access and provision of care to children and families.

- Demonstrates an understanding of the laws that impact confidentiality in the provision of care (e.g., Health Insurance Portability Accountability Act [HIPAA] and Family Educational Rights and Privacy Act [FERPA]).

- Advocates for children and parents to assure they are afforded the rights guaranteed to them by federal law (e.g., Individuals with Disabilities Education Act [IDEA]).

Additional measurement criteria for the Advanced Practice Pediatric Nurse:

The Advanced Practice Pediatric Nurse:

- Advances the profession through enhancing public awareness and health professional familiarity with the advanced practice pediatric nursing role and scope of practice.

REFERENCES

Alexander, J.E. et al. (1998). Virginia Henderson: Definition of nursing. In A. Tomey & Alligood, M. (Eds.), *Nursing theorists and their work* (4th ed., pp. 99–111). St. Louis: Mosby.

American Association of Colleges of Nursing. (1996). *The essentials of master's education for advanced practice nursing.* Washington, DC: AACN.

American Association of Colleges of Nursing. (1998). *The essentials of baccalaureate education for professional nursing practice.* Washington, DC: AACN.

American Association of Colleges of Nursing. (2006). *The essentials of doctoral education for advanced nursing practice.* Washington, DC: AACN.

American Nurses Association. (2001). *Code of ethics for nurses with interpretive statements.* Silver Spring, MD: Nursesbooks.org.

American Nurses Association. (2003). *Nursing's social policy statement* (2nd ed.). Silver Spring, MD: Nursesbooks.org.

American Nurses Association. (2004). *Nursing: Scope and standards of practice.* Silver Spring, MD: Nursesbooks.org.

American Nurses Association & Society of Pediatric Nurses. (2003). *Scope and standards of pediatric nursing practice.* Silver Spring, MD: Nursesbooks.org.

American Public Health Association, Inc. (1955). *Health supervision of young children.* New York, NY: APHA.

Association of Camp Nurses. (2005). *The scope and standards of camp nursing practice* (2nd ed.). Bernidji, MN: Association of Camp Nurses.

Association of Social Work Boards (ASWB), Federation of State Boards of Physical Therapy (FSBPT), Federation of State Medical Boards (FSMB), National Board for Certification in Occupational Therapy (NMCOT), National Council of State Boards of Nursing, Inc. (NCSBN), & the National Association of Boards of Pharmacy (NABP). (2007). *Changes in healthcare professions' scope of practice: Legislative considerations*. Retrieved April 19, 2008, from https://www.ncsbn.org/ScopeofPractice.pdf

Betz, C. L. (2003). Nurse's role in promoting health transitions for adolescents and young adults with developmental disabilities. *Nursing Clinics of North America, 38*(2), 271–89.

Betz, C.L. (2004a). Transition of adolescents with special health care needs: Review and analysis of the literature. *Issues in Comprehensive Pediatric Nursing, 27*, 179–241.

Betz, C. L. (2004b). Adolescents in transition of adult care: Why the concern? *Nursing Clinics of North America*, 39(4), 681–713.

Brady, N. & Lewin, L. (2007). Evidence-based practice in nursing: Bridging the gap between research and practice. *Journal of Pediatric Health Care, 21*, 53–56.

Breuner, C.C., Barry, P.J., & Kemper, K.J. (1998). Alternative medicine by homeless youth. *Archives Pediatric Adolescent Medicine, 152*, 1071–1075.

Caplan, G. (1961). *An approach to community mental health*. New York, NY: Grune and Stratton.

Children's Defense Fund. (2006). *Improving children's health: Understanding children's health disparities and promising approaches to address them*. Washington, DC: CDF.

Connolly, C. (2005). Growth and development of a specialty: The professionalization of child health care. *Pediatric Nursing, 31*, 211–215.

Consensus Panel on Genetic/Genomic Nursing Competencies. (2006). *Essential nursing competencies and curricula guidelines for genetics and genomics*. Silver Spring, MD: American Nurses Association.

Cowell, J. & Swartwout, K. (2006). Healthcare home: Ensuring access to a regular healthcare provider. In M. Craft-Rosenberg and M. Krajicek (Eds.), *Nursing excellence for children and families* (pp. 23–40). New York, NY: Springer Publishing Co.

Craft-Rosenberg, M. & Krajicek, M. (2006). *Nursing excellence for children and families*. New York, NY: Springer Publishing Co.

Crowley, A. (2001). Child care health consultation: An ecological model. *Journal of the Society of Pediatric Nurses, 6* (4), 170–181.

Deatrick, J. (2006). Family partnerships in nursing care. In M. Craft-Rosenberg and Krajicek, M. (Eds.), *Nursing excellence for children and families* (pp. 41–56). New York, NY: Springer Publishing Co.

Deatrick, J. & Knafl, K. (1990). Management behaviors: Day-to-day adjustments to childhood chronic conditions. *Journal of Pediatric Nursing, 5,* 15–22.

Duderstadt, K., Hughes, K., Soobader, M., & Newacheck, P. (2006). The impact of public insurance expansions on children's access and use of care. *Pediatrics, 118* (4), 1676–1682.

Field, M.J. & Behrman, R.E. (Eds.), (2003). *When children die: Improving palliative and end-of-life are for children and their families.* Institute of Medicine of the National Academies. Washington, DC: National Academies Press.

Gance-Cleveland, B. (2001). Pediatric nurses: Advocates against youth violence. *Journal of the Society of Pediatric Nurses, 6* (3), 133–142.

Gance-Cleveland, B., Costin, D.K. & Degenstein, J.A. (2003). School-based health centers: Statewide quality improvement program. *Journal of Nursing Care Quality, 18*(4), 288–94.

Guilday, P. (2000). School nursing practice today: Implications for the future. *Journal of School Nursing, 16*(5), 25–31.

Harrison, T.W. (2003). Adolescent homosexuality and concerns regarding disclosure. *Journal of School Health, 73* (3), 107–112.

Henderson, V. (1964). The nature of nursing. *American Journal of Nursing, 64*(8), 62–68.

Institute of Medicine. (2001). *Crossing the quality chasm: A new health system for the 21st century*. Washington, DC: National Academy of Sciences.

Knafl, K., Breitmayer, B., Gallo, A., & Zoeller, L. (1996). Family response to childhood chronic illness: Description of management styles. *Journal of Pediatric Nursing, 11*, 315–326.

Knafl, K. & Deatrick, J. (2002). The challenge of normalization for families of children with chronic conditions. *Pediatric Nursing, 28*, 48–56.

Lewandowski, L. & Tesler, M. (2003). *Family-centered care: Putting it into action – the SPN/ANA guide to family-centered care*. Washington, DC: Nursesbooks.org.

Melynk, B. & Fineout-Overholt, E. (Ed.), (2005). *Evidence-based practice in nursing and health care*. Philadelphia, PA: Lippincott, Williams and Wilkins.

Melnyk, B. & Moldenhauer, Z. (2006). *The KySSSM guide to child and adolescent mental health screening, early intervention and health promotion*. Cherry Hill, NJ: National Association of Pediatric Nurse Practitioners.

Miles, M.S. (1996). News from the society: A historical perspective. *Journal of the Society of Pediatric Nurses, 1*(1), 46–47.

Murphy, M. (1990). A brief history of pediatric nurse practitioners and NAPNAP: 1964–1990. *Journal of Pediatric Health Care, 4*, 332–338.

National Association of Children's Hospitals and Related Institutions. (2006). *All children need children's hospitals*. Retrieved April 19, 2008, from http://www.childrenshospitals.net/AM/Template.cfm?Section=Fact_Sheet&Template=/TaggedPage/TaggedPageDisplay.cfm&TPLID=61&ContentID=2262.

National Association of Clinical Nurse Specialists. (2004). *Statement on clinical nurse specialist practice and education.* (2nd ed.). Harrisburg, PA: NACNS.

National Association of Neonatal Nurses. (2006). *Education standards for neonatal nurse practitioner programs.* Glenview, IL: NANN. Retrieved May 29, 2008, from http://www.nann.org/pdf/NNP_Standards.pdf National Association of Pediatric Nurse Practitioners. (2002a). NAPNAP position statement on age parameters for PNP practice. *Journal of Pediatric Health Care, 16,* A36.

National Association of Pediatric Nurse Practitioners. (2002b). NAPNAP position statement on the pediatric health care home. *Journal of Pediatric Health Care, 17,* A22.

National Association of Pediatric Nurse Practitioners. (2004a). NAPNAP position statement on protection of children involved in research studies. *Journal of Pediatric Health Care, 18,* A20–A21.

National Association of Pediatric Nurse Practitioners. (2004b). *Scope and standards of practice: Pediatric nurse practitioner (PNP).* Cherry Hill, NJ: NAPNAP.

National Association of Pediatric Nurse Practitioners. (2005a). NAPNAP position statement on the acute care nurse practitioner. *Journal of Pediatric Health Care, 19,* A38–A39.

National Association of Pediatric Nurse Practitioners. (2005b). NAPNAP position statement on school-based and school-linked centers. *Journal of Pediatric Health Care, 19,* A25–A26

National Association of Pediatric Nurse Practitioners. (2006a). NAPNAP position statement on health risks and needs of gay, lesbian, bisexual, transgender and questioning (GLBTQ) adolescents. *Journal of Pediatric Health Care, 20,* A29–A30.

National Association of Pediatric Nurse Practitioners. (2006b). *Healthy Eating and Activity Together (HEAT^{TM}) clinical practice guideline: Identifying and preventing overweight in childhood.* Cherry Hill, NJ: NAPNP.

National Association of Pediatric Nurse Practitioners. (2007). NAPNAP position statement on access to care. *Journal of Pediatric Health Care, 21,* A35–A36.

National Association of School Nurses. (2002). *Position statement: Education, licensure, and certification of school nurses.* Retrieved April 19, 2008, from http://www.nasn.org/Portals/0/positions/2002pseducation.pdf

National Association of School Nurses. (2003). *Access to a school nurse.* Retrieved May 29, 2008, from http://www.nasn.org/Portals/0/statements/resolutionaccess.pdf

National Association of School Nurses. (2006). *School nursing management of students with chronic health conditions.* Scarborough, ME: NASN. Retrieved June 27, 2007, from: http://www.nasn.org/Default.aspx?tabid=351

National Association of School Nurses & American Nurses Association. (2005). *School nursing: Scope and standards of practice.* Silver Spring, MD: Nursesbooks.org.

National Center for Complementary and Alternative Medicine (NCCAM). (2007). *CAM basics.* Retrieved April 19, 2008, from http://nccam.nih.gov/health/whatiscam/.

National Organization of Nurse Practitioner Faculties. (2006a). *Domains and core competencies of nurse practitioner practice.* Washington, DC: NONPF.

National Organization of Nurse Practitioner Faculties. (2006b). *Advanced nursing practice: Curriculum guidelines and program standards for nurse practitioner education.* Washington, DC: NONPF.

National Panel for Acute Care Nurse Practitioner Competencies. (2004). *Acute care nurse practitioner competencies.* Washington, DC: NONPF.

Nehring, W. M., Roth, S. P., Natvig, D., Betz, C. L., Savage, T., & Krajicek, M. (2004). *Intellectual and developmental disabilities nursing: Scope and standards of practice.* American Nurses Association and the American Association on Mental Retardation. Washington, DC: Nursesbooks.org.

Nelson, J. (2003). Providing health care to lesbian, gay, bisexual and transgender adolescents. In D.A. Gaffney & C. Roye (Eds.), *Adolescent Sexual Development and Sexuality.* Kingston, NJ: Civic Research Institute, Inc.

Ottolini, M., Hamburger, E., Loprieto, J., Coleman, R.H., Sachs, H.C., Madden, R., & Brasseux, C. (1999, May). *Alternative medicine use among children in the Washington, DC, area.* Paper presented at the meeting of the Pediatric Academic Societies. San Francisco, CA.

Pearson, L. (2007). The Pearson Report: A national overview of nurse practitioner legislation and healthcare issues. *American Journal for Nurse Practitioners, 11*(2), 10–101.

Percy, M. & Sperhac, A. (2007). State regulations for the pediatric nurse practitioner in acute care. *Journal of Pediatric Health Care, 21* (1), 29–43.

Plotnick, J. (2007, March). *Responding globally to the world's children: Addressing health care needs.* Symposium conducted at the annual meeting of the National Association of Pediatric Nurse Practitioners. Lake Buena Vista, FL.

Pridham, K. F. (1993). Anticipatory guidance of parents of new infants: Potential contribution of the internal working model construct. *Image: Journal of Nursing Scholarship, 25,* 49–56.

Ramler, M., Nakatsukasa-Ono., W., Loe, C. & Harris, K. (2006). *The influence of child care health consultants in promoting children's health and well-being: A report on selected resources.* Retrieved April 19, 2008, from http://hcccnsc.edc.org/resources/data/CC_lit_review_Screen_All.pdf

Sackett, D.L., Straus, S.E., Richardson, W.S., Rosenberg, W., & Haynes, R. B. (2000). *Evidence-based medicine: How to practice and teach EBM.* Edinburgh, UK: Churchill Livingstone.

Safriet, B.J. (1992). Health care dollars and regulatory sense: The role of advanced practice nursing. *Yale Journal on Regulation, 9*(2), 417–488.

Safriet, B.J. (2002). Closing the gap between *can* and *may* in health-care providers' scopes of practice: A primer for policymakers. *Yale Journal on Regulation, 19*: 301–334.

Shelton, T. L. & Sepanek, J. S. (1994). *Family-centered care for children needing specialized health and developmental services.* Bethesda, MD: Association for the Care of Children's Health.

Society of Pediatric Nurses. (2004). *The role of the staff nurse in protecting children and families involved in research.* Retrieved April 19, 2008, from https://www.pedsnurses.org/index.php?option=com_docman &task=doc_view&gid=68&Itemid=117.

Sullivan, E.J. (2004). *Becoming influential: A guide for nurses.* Upper Saddle River, NJ: Pearson Education, Inc.

Taylor, M. (2006). Mapping the literature of pediatric nursing. *Journal of the Medical Library Association 94* (Suppl. 2), E-128–E-136.

U.S. Department of Health and Human Services. (2002). *Children's health highlights.* (AHRQ Publication No. 02-P005).

U.S. Department of Health and Human Services. (2005). *Selected findings on child and adolescent health care hrom the 2004 National Healthcare Quality/Disparities Reports.* (AHRQ Publication No. 05-P011).

Woodring, B. C. & Pridham, K.F. (Ed.), (1998). *Standards and guidelines for pre-licensure and early professional education for the nursing care of children and their families. (Revised).* Department of Health and Human Services, Bureau of Maternal and Child Health, Document #H112R77. Washington, DC: U.S. Government Printing Office.

World Health Organization. (2007). *International classification of functioning, disability and health—Children and youth version (ICF–CY).* Geneva: WHO.

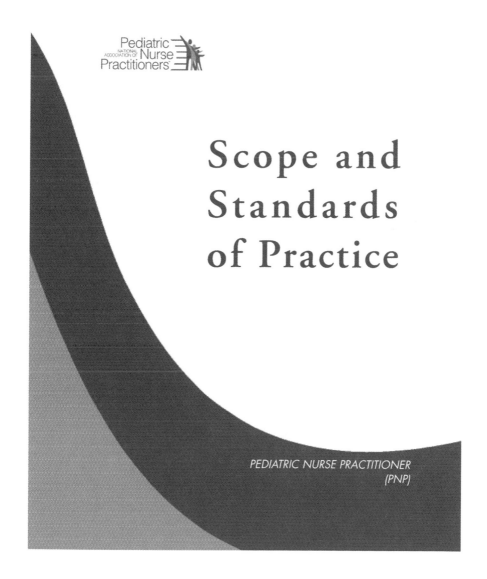

Scope and
Standards
of Practice

PEDIATRIC NURSE PRACTITIONER
(PNP)

SCOPE AND STANDARDS OF PRACTICE:
PEDIATRIC NURSE PRACTITIONER (PNP)

SCOPE OF PRACTICE

Definition

The Pediatric Nurse Practitioner (PNP) is an advanced practice registered nurse who provides health care to children from birth through 21 years of age, and in specific situations, to individuals older than the age of 21 years. To function in this role, the PNP must have completed a formal educational program specializing in pediatric health care and have met the State Board's regulations that govern advanced practice nursing.

Education

Current entry-level preparation for pediatric nurse practitioner practice is a master's degree in nursing science. The educational focus of PNP programs is on the care of children, professional leadership, research utilization for evidence-based practice, consultation, advocacy, and systems intervention to enhance care quality. The curricular content includes growth and development; pathophysiology; pharmacology; health promotion; ethics; physical, developmental, family, cultural, community, and environmental assessment; laboratory skills; and the diagnosis and management of behavioral problems and childhood illnesses, both acute and chronic conditions. The curriculum includes didactic and clinical practice components.

Practice Parameters

PNPs are pediatric health care professionals who provide comprehensive health care to children through assessment, diagnosis, management, and evaluation of care. In accordance with state licensure and regulatory mechanisms, PNPs provide a wide range of pediatric health care services in a variety of health care settings. The PNP may consult with other members of the health care team, may coordinate care, and/or make referrals to other members of the health care team. Additionally, the PNP may function as a consultant to nurse practitioner colleagues and other disciplines in areas of expertise. The professional role of the PNP's practice requires the PNP to assume accountability for professional actions, including incorporating risk management strategies into clinical practice.

PNPs practice under their state Nurse Practice Act and in accordance with individual state laws and regulations. Since all fifty (50) states vary in their regulations as to the definition, scope of practice, and prescriptive authority of nurse practitioners, specific state requirements for practice must be identified and met. Prescription of appropriate pharmacological agents is an essential and necessary component of comprehensive management by PNPs.

STANDARDS OF PRACTICE

Process of Care

The PNP uses a framework for practice that incorporates both scientific and theoretical bases. The scope of health care services and standards of practice provided by PNPs are impacted by state Nurse Practice Acts, licensure and regulatory mechanisms, work setting privileges and/or credentialing, and collaborative agreements, where necessary. The scope of health care services and standards of practice provided by PNPs include, but are not limited to, the following:

Assessment and Diagnosis:

• Obtain a comprehensive developmental, health, and medical history

- Perform physical examinations based on age and history
- Order and interpret age-appropriate and condition-specific screening tests, laboratory tests, and diagnostic procedures
- Systematically compare and contrast clinical findings in formulating differential diagnoses
- Assess and diagnose childhood illnesses, including chronic and acute conditions, or any other condition that is within the expertise and knowledge of the PNP
- Formulate a holistic, culturally sensitive, family-centered plan of care in collaboration with the child and family as active participants
- Consult with other health care providers as necessary

Interventions:

- Provide comprehensive health plans by teaching, counseling, and advising children and their families about growth and development, health promotion, health status, illnesses, illness management plans, as well as providing anticipatory guidance
- Treat childhood illnesses, chronic and acute conditions, or any other condition that is within the scope of practice, expertise, and knowledge of the PNP
- Involve family/child in decision-making regarding plan of care and responsibilities
- Prescribe/order appropriate pharmacological and nonpharmacological interventions, including complementary and alternative therapies (within limits of state-legislated prescriptive authority and knowledge of the PNP)
- Provide appropriate child and family education regarding purpose, regimens, side effects, possible interactions of medications and/or treatments, cost, and alternative treatments or procedures
- Provide for appropriate follow-up care
- Utilize any other appropriate intervention(s) within the scope of practice parameters, expertise, and knowledge of the PNP

- Provide care that reflects evidence-based practice
- Provide care that reflects consideration of ethical implications, cost and clinical effectiveness, and family acceptance/satisfaction
- Consult and collaborate with other health care providers as appropriate
- Coordinate care, make appropriate referrals, and facilitate health systems intervention to assure quality care
- Identify and coordinate access to appropriate community resources
- Advocate for children and their families
- Provide care that is culturally competent and family centered

Evaluation:

- Monitor and evaluate accuracy of diagnosis and effectiveness of prescribed treatment plans, growth, and development
- Monitor child and family response to treatments
- Modify interventions based on effectiveness, available evidence-based practice guidelines, and individual child and family needs/satisfaction
- Systematically monitor effectiveness of practice through client database and outcomes evaluation
- Participate in Continuous Quality Improvement processes to assure provision of quality health care
- Synthesize and use the results of evaluation to make or recommend changes including policy, procedure, or protocol documentation

Collaborative Responsibilities

As part of the interdisciplinary team:

- Partner with other disciplines to enhance care through activities such as education, consultation, collaboration, development of new management and therapeutic strategies, or research

This appendix is not current and is of historical significance only.

- Model expert practice to interdisciplinary team members and families

- Function in a variety of roles such as health care provider, consultant, educator, researcher, and administrator

Professional Accountability

As health care professionals:

- Demonstrate practice consistent with legal standards in compliance with any applicable state and federal regulations

- Work to influence policy-making bodies to improve care

- Support the education and role development of novice practitioners by serving as preceptors, role models, and mentors

- Use an ethical framework to evaluate issues regarding care

- Maintain active membership in professional organizations

- Demonstrate practice consistent with professional standards, including current NAPNAP and State Board of Registered Nursing regulations for advanced nurse practitioners

- Maintain appropriate malpractice coverage

- Advance the profession through enhancing public awareness and health professional familiarity with the PNP role and scope of practice

Continued Competence

Emphasizing the importance of ongoing continuing education:

- Maintain clinical competency, professional skills, and knowledge through experiences and formal continuing education programs and independent learning activities

- Evaluate the practice environment and quality of nursing care provided in relation to existing evidence, identifying opportunities for the generation and use of research

- Seek feedback and evaluation of one's own practice

- Meet and maintain eligibility for national and/or state certification programs

Quality Assurance

Recognizing the need for ongoing quality improvement:

- Initiate and revise protocols or guidelines to reflect accepted changes in care management or to address emerging problems

- Modify practice consistent with current practice guidelines and clinical recommendations for the health care of children in all settings, including but not limited to primary, acute, critical, long-term, and chronic care settings

Adopted by the National Association of Pediatric Nurse Practitioners' Executive Board on January 22, 2004

©2004 National Association of Pediatric Nurse Practitioners. Cherry Hill, NJ. All rights reserved.

The purpose of this document is to define the Scope and Standards of Practice for Pediatric Nurse Practitioners. It replaces the following documents: *Scope of Practice for Pediatric Nurse Practitioners in Primary Care*, ©2000, National Association of Pediatric Nurse Practitioners and *Standards of Practice for Pediatric Nurse Practitioners*, ©2001, Association of Faculty of Pediatric Nurse Practitioner Programs and National Association of Pediatric Nurse Practitioners.

Acknowledgments
The National Association of Pediatric Nurse Practitioners would like to acknowledge the contribution of the following individuals from the NAPNAP Scope and Standards of Practice Task Force:

Patricia Jackson Allen, MSN, RN, CS, PNP, FAAN (Chair)
Melanie Percy, PhD, CPNP
Dolores Jones, EdD, CPNP
Catherine Goodhue, MSN, RN, CPNP
Holly Lieder, CPNP
Patricia Thompson, MS, CPNP
Keli Hansen, MS, CPNP
Sara Majors, BSN

Supporting Organization
The following organization has supported the National Association of Pediatric Nurse Practitioners' *Scope and Standards for Pediatric Nurse Practitioners*.
Association of Faculties of Pediatric Nurse Practitioners, January 30, 2004

APPENDIX B
SCOPE AND STANDARDS OF
PEDIATRIC NURSING PRACTICE
(2003)

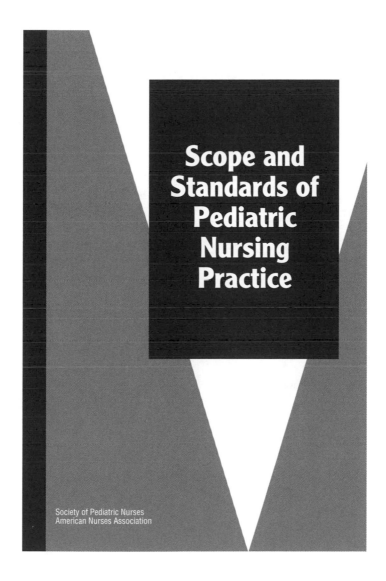

Scope and
Standards of
Pediatric
Nursing
Practice

Society of Pediatric Nurses
American Nurses Association

This appendix is not current and is of historical significance only.

Library of Congress Cataloging-in-Publication Data

Family-centered care : putting it into action : the SPN/ANA guide to family-centered care.
    p. ; cm.
    ISBN 1-55810-210-8
    1. Pediatric nursing. 2. Family nursing.
    [DNLM: 1. Family—psychology. 2. Family Nursing. 3. Professional-Family Relations. 4. Sibling Relations. WY 159.5 F198 2003] I. Title: SPN/ANA guide to family-centered care. II. Society of Pediatric Nurses. III. American Nurses Association.

    RJ245.F35 2003
    610.73'62—dc21

2003006966

Published by
nursesbooks.org
The Publishing Program of ANA
American Nurses Association
600 Maryland Avenue, SW
Suite 100 West
Washington, D.C. 20024-2571

ISBN 1-55810-210-8

PNP23   2.5M   06/03

This appendix is not current and is of historical significance only.

Acknowledgements

Society of Pediatric Nurses Practice Standards Nursing Task Force...

...for Revision of the Basic Practice Scope and Standards
Vicky R. Bowden, DNSc, RN, CPN
Mary Markov, MS Ed, RN, CPN
Michele Mendes, PhD, RN
Rosemary McLaughlin, MSN, RN
Wayne Neal, RN

...for Development of the Advanced Practice Scope and Standards
Janet Deatrick, PhD, RN, FAAN, Chair
Cathy Bartolone, MSN, RN
Marion Broome, PhD, RN, FAAN
Martha A. Q. Curley, PhD, RN, CCNS, FAAN
Barbara Durand, EdD, RN, FAAN
Lois Linden, MS, RN
Margaret Miles, PhD, RN, FAAN
Mary T. Perkins, PhD, RN
Marilyn Savedra, PhD, RN, FAAN
Judy Verger, MSN, RN
Barbara Woodring, EdD, RN

In addition, the following SPN members assisted with review and editing of the final document:
Vicky Bowden, DNSc, RN
Carol Shega Kline, MSN, RN
Anne Marie Kotzer, PhD, RN
Linda Lewandowksi, PhD, RN
Maura McPhee, PhD, RN

ANA Staff
Carol Bickford, MS, RN, C
Winifred Carson, JD
Yvonne Humes, BBA

PREFACE

Pediatric nursing historically has not had national or international standards of care or education. While often merged with other specialties within nursing, such as *maternal*-child or *parent*-child nursing, no succinct guidelines are available to pediatric nurses who work in practice or educational settings. As the theoretical, practice, and research bases for pediatric nursing matured, the need for standards of practice for all pediatric nurses, including pediatric advanced practice registered nurses, became evident.[1] At the same time, other organizations challenged advanced practice nursing to clarify standards of education, practice, and certification.[2] This set of circumstances provided the Society of Pediatric Nurses (SPN) with an opportunity to create standards of practice that are congruent with current professional policy for both the nurse generalist and the advanced practice nurse.

In 1993, SPN established an Advanced Practice Task Force, with members from the Education and Clinical Practice Committees, to provide guidance to the Board of Directors related to developing vision and support for the roles of the Advanced Practice Pediatric Registered Nurse. Among the topics addressed were the development of Standards for Advanced Practice and publication of *Scope and Standards for the Advanced Practice Pediatric Nurse*. Guidelines were also developed for educating Advanced Practice Pediatric Nurses and are included as an appendix to this document.

The American Nurses Association (ANA) created the Council on Advanced Practice Nursing to address common issues and goals among advanced practice nurses in diverse settings. The ANA Social Policy statement[3, 4] was updated to clarify that master's prepared nurse practitioners and clinical nurse specialists whose clinical practice reflects specialization, expansion, and advancement are included with those who are considered advanced practice nurses. The *Scope and Standards of Advanced Practice Registered Nursing*[1], which serves as the framework for these pediatric advanced practice standards, was also developed. Most recently, ANA's Congress on Nursing Practice and Economics approved revised criteria for scopes of nursing practice and revised criteria for designation of areas of specialty practice.[5]

ANA and SPN jointly published *Statement on the Scope and Standards of Pediatric Clinical Nursing Practice* in 1996, which focused on the standards of nursing care and professional performance for pediatric nurses. The current revision incorporates major changes to address the expanded scope of practice that represents the specialty of pediatric nursing and to include the additional standards of practice and professional performance for the advanced practice pediatric nurse.

CONTENTS

Preface   **92**
Introduction   **97**
    Family-Centered Care   98
    Practice Context   100

Scope of Practice for Pediatric Nursing   **103**
    Levels of Pediatric Nursing Practice   103
        The Pediatric Nurse—Generalist Level   103
        The Advanced Practice Pediatric Nurse   104
        Key Elements and Defining Characteristics
          of the Advanced Practice Nurse   108
    Settings for Pediatric Nursing Practice   110
        Inpatient Setting   110
        Outpatient Clinics and Offices   111
        Community Health Care   112
        Home Health Care   112
        School Settings   113
        Air and Surface Transport   114
        Camp Settings   115
    Education   116
    Certification   117
    Regulation   118

Standards of Pediatric Nursing Practice   **119**
    Definition and Role of Standards   119
    Development of Standards   119
    Assumptions   120
    Organizing Principles of the Scope and Standards   120
      of Pediatric Nursing Practice
    Standards of Care   122
    Standards of Professional Performance   123
    Criteria   123
    Guidelines   124
    Summary   124

Standards of Care   127

    Standard 1. Assessment   127
    Standard 2. Diagnosis   129
    Standard 3. Outcome Identification   130
    Standard 4. Planning   132
    Standard 5. Implementation   133
        5a. Case Management and Coordination   134
            of Comprehensive Health Services
        5b. Consultation   135
        5c. Health Promotion, Health Maintenance, and 136
            Health Teaching
        5d. Prescriptive Authority   136
        5e. Referral   138
    Standard 6. Evaluation   108

Standards of Professional Performance   139

    Standard 1. Quality of Care   139
    Standard 2. Performance Appraisal   141
    Standard 3. Education   142
    Standard 4. Collegiality   142
    Standard 5. Ethics   143
    Standard 6. Collaboration   145
    Standard 7. Research   146
    Standard 8. Resource Utilization   147

Glossary   148
References   155
Appendix: Guidelines for APP RN Education   161

    Background   161
    Education and Practice   162
    Course Work and Clinical Experience   162
    Faculty   164
    Areas of Curricular Focus and Competencies   165

INTRODUCTION

Scope and Standards of Pediatric Nursing Practice is intended to be used in conjunction with *Standards and Guidelines for Pre-licensure and Professional Education for the Nursing Care of Children and Their Families*[6-7] and other documents that outline the values, beliefs, and practice of pediatric nurses. *Scope and Standards of Pediatric Nursing Practice* guides the practice of nurses in generalist or advanced practice roles who provide services to children and their families. It may also be useful to families and other stakeholders such as administrators, educators, policy makers, and others paying for health care.

The age of children seen by pediatric health practitioners ranges from neonates (less than one month old, including those gestationally premature) to adolescents in their late teens. Healthcare professionals also recognize that care of the child must extend to care of the family and its needs in relation to optimizing the growth and development of the child. The child is an integral entity within the family constellation. The child cannot be viewed as separate and apart from the group of individuals who play such an influential role in molding the child's behavior, emotions, and understanding of the world. Thus, the focus of pediatric nursing is the child *and* the family. The philosophy of care that has been adopted in pediatric nursing is aptly called *family-centered care.*

Because it is no longer possible to define the family in strict terms of the composition of its members or within the context of its previously defined functions, broader definitions of the family have emerged that conceptualize the family without the boundaries previously respected by the law and by societal sanctions.[8] In the most general sense, a family today is defined as "two or more people joined together by bonds of sharing and intimacy."[9] Within this constellation of members, the functions of the family are to provide "for the physical and health needs of its members, serve as a locus of love, intimacy, and motivation, and provide sociologic, cultural, and psychologic roots."[10] Although these definitions do not fit those stipulated by the law or many religious institutions, when the health and well-being of a loved one is at risk, legal and religious boundaries cannot serve as the sole inclusion criteria for family-centered healthcare interventions.

At the same time, the healthcare providers' actions cannot overlook the familial connections that are legally sanctioned and need to be recognized when the healthcare issues of a child are in question. Bozett suggested that the most workable definition of the family is this: the family is who the patient says it is.[10] This definition frees the nurse from value judgments about the importance of certain familial ties within a given family and allows for practices and policies to be instituted that are in the best interest of the child.

Family-Centered Care

Family-centered care is a philosophy of care that acknowledges the importance of the family unit as the fundamental focus of all healthcare interventions. This model of care recognizes that the family is central in a child's life and should be central in the child's plan of care.[11] The Association for the Care of Children's Health (ACCH) has recognized that the term family-centered care cannot simply be described by a common definition. Rather, extracting and explaining the elements or components of this philosophy of care, which work together to move an individual or an institution toward providing a family-centered approach, best explain family-centered care.

Eight elements have been defined, each serving to reinforce, facilitate, and complement the implementation of the others (see Table 1). The elements of family-centered care recognize each family's uniqueness, acknowledge the influence of the family as a constant in the child's life, and emphasize the importance of providing services which demonstrate the value of collaboration between the healthcare provider, the child, and the family. Family-centered care is based on the premise that a positive adjustment to a child's level of health and well-being requires the involvement of the whole family. [12]

Family-Centered Care: Putting it into Action—The SPN/ANA Guide to Family-Centered Care[64] further expands upon these elements and provides evidence-based practice recommendations that more fully describe this practice model.

Table 1: *Key Elements of Family-Centered Care*

Care Element	Description
Element 1: The Family at the Center	Incorporate into policy and practice the recognition that the family is the constant in a child's life, while the service systems and support personnel within those systems fluctuate and that the illness or injury of a child affects all members of the family.
Element 2: Family–Professional Collaboration	Facilitate family–professional collaboration at all levels of hospital, home, and community care for: • care of an individual child; • program development, implementation, evaluation, and evolution, and • policy formation.
Element 3: Family–Professional Communication	Exchange complete and unbiased information between families and professionals in a supportive manner at all times.
Element 4: Cultural Diversity of Families	Incorporate into policy and practice the recognition and honoring of cultural diversity, strengths, and individuality within and across all families, including ethnic, racial, spiritual, social, economic, educational, and geographic diversity.
Element 5: Coping Differences and Supports	Recognize and respect different methods of coping and implement comprehensive policies and programs that provide families with the developmental, educational, emotional, spiritual, environmental, and financial supports needed to meet their diverse needs.
Element 6: Family-Centered Peer Support	Encourage and facilitate family-to-family support and networking.
Element 7: Specialized Service and Support Systems	Ensure that hospital, home, and community service and support systems for children needing specialized health and developmental care and their families are flexible, accessible, and comprehensive in responding to diverse family-identified needs.
Element 8: Holistic Perspective of Family-Centered Care	Appreciate families as families and children as children, recognizing that they possess a wide range of strengths, concerns, emotions, and aspirations beyond their need for specialized health and developmental services and support.

Practice Context

As a whole, child health has improved over the past 25 years in areas such as infant mortality and preventable childhood illnesses. However, some 30% of all U.S. children have serious, chronic healthcare needs and some 10% of those have severe conditions and often have two or more conditions that use 25% of the child healthcare dollars.[13-14] Chronically ill children are a diverse group having over 3700 different chronic conditions. The most common conditions are respiratory disorders, musculoskeletal disorders, and attention deficit disorders.[15] In 2000, 7% of children between the ages of 5 and 17 and 34% of children younger than 5 were limited in their activities because of one or more chronic conditions.[16] 90% of children with serious healthcare needs now survive into adulthood. Children's healthcare needs are all exacerbated by social, economic, family, and psychological issues, as well as by a fragmented and culturally biased healthcare system.[13-14]

In 1993, the poverty rate for children living with family members reached a high of 22% of the child population. In 2000, 16% of children lived in families with income below the poverty threshold. Children in families below the poverty line were nearly three times more likely to experience food insecurity and hunger than those children in families with incomes above poverty level. Children living in poverty tend to be in poorer health than children in higher income families; however, it has been noted that the health gap between children below and those at or above poverty level has decreased slightly between 1994 and 2000.[16]

The child death rate, while decreasing over the previous decade, claimed the lives of 35 per 100,000 for children ages 1 to 4, and 19 per 100,000 for children ages 5 to 14 in 1999.[16] The decrease is attributed to advances in medical care and fewer deaths by motor vehicle accidents. However, healthcare providers continue to be challenged to provide accessible care to lower the death rate. Black children continue to have the highest death rates while Asian/Pacific Islander children have the lowest death rate.[16] Unintentional injuries are the leading cause of death in all age ranges (1 to 14). Use of child restraint systems (including safety seats, booster seats, and seat belts) are credited for reducing the number and severity of injuries to children in motor vehicles. In 1999, 47% of child occupants ages 1 to 4 who died in automobile accidents were unrestrained. Other major causes of death include birth defects, cancer, and homicides (in older children). Death rates of adolescents (age 15 to 19) are 70 per 100,000. Homicide, suicide, and unintentional injuries continue to account for over 3 out of 4 deaths in this age group. Injuries from motor vehicle and firearm accidents are the primary causes of death.[16-17]

Teen birth rates are associated with increased risk for low birth weight. While the rates for teen births rose during the mid-1980s and early 1990s, they have declined steadily in the past several years.16 However, for those teens and families involved, teenage childbirth may result in fewer opportunities, lower education, and increased likelihood of living in poverty for both mother and child; thus, increasing the chances for poorer health outcomes.

More than 11 million American children lack health insurance today to pay for health care. 90% of these children have parents who work. The State Children's Health Insurance Program (SCHIP), which was passed in 1997, has expanded Medicaid to cover uninsured children with family income above current eligibility levels but too low to afford private health insurance. Despite this insurance program, healthcare insurance coverage for children remains in need of further expansion to cover the many children left uninsured.[18]

Over the years, nursing has gained knowledge and expertise that is now being applied in generalist and advanced practice nursing and tested in research. Certainly, pediatric nursing on both the generalist and advanced levels has much to contribute to the provision of services to children's healthcare needs. Advanced Practice Registered Nurse (APRN) care has been shown to be cost-efficient and high in quality,[19-22] and applicable to children who are medically complex, such as those with HIV-related diseases.[23] All Advanced Practice Registered Nurses need to be appropriately reimbursed for care. Such reimbursement varies among the advanced practice roles and is determined by individual state regulations and third-party reimbursers.[24-25] Educating all pediatric nurses to care for children's primary healthcare needs and to care for children with special healthcare needs will contribute to the overall care of children whose situations place them at risk for increased vulnerability.

SCOPE OF PRACTICE FOR PEDIATRIC NURSING

The scope of practice and roles of the pediatric nurse are diverse and dynamic. The intention of this document is to explore some of the current issues and trends to define current roles and the potential for new or convergent roles to meet the ever-changing healthcare needs of children and their families in a variety of settings. The document is not intended to restrict role development, but rather to clarify the scope and foundation of generalist and advanced practice pediatric nursing, and to distinguish between these levels of practice.

Levels of Pediatric Nursing Practice

Pediatric nurses are licensed registered nurses practicing on either the generalist or advanced level. These levels of practice are described below.

The Pediatric Nurse—Generalist Level

The pediatric nurse who practices on the *generalist* level is a licensed registered nurse who has demonstrated clinical skills and knowledge within the specialty. Many nurses contribute to the care of children and their families and are also responsible for adhering to the specialty practice standards as designated by the profession.

In 1998 the Society of Pediatric Nursing (SPN) completed a project funded by the Health Resources and Services Administration (HRSA) Maternal and Child Health Bureau that identified standards for pediatric pre-licensure and early professional development.[6-7] While these concepts and competencies apply to the education of the beginning practitioner, they offer a unique description of the boundaries of pediatric nursing on a generalist level including:

- The unique anatomical, physiological, and developmental differences among neonates, infants, children, and adolescents;
- Care of children in the context of their families;

- Sensitivity to cultural issues, especially those related to how the family and healthcare providers tend to children's healthcare needs;

- Communicating effectively with children, families, and other healthcare providers;

- Safety assurance and injury prevention for children and their families;

- Promotion of children's health in the context of their families;

- Needs unique to the growth and development of children who have chronic conditions, and their families;

- Exceptional needs of children with episodic injuries or illnesses;

- Economic, social, and political influences outside the family that have an impact on children's health and development and family functioning; and

- Ethical, moral, and legal dilemmas involving children, families, and healthcare professionals.

The Advanced Practice Pediatric Nurse

The pediatric nurse who practices on the *advanced* level has a master's degree, specializing and expanding their role through formal education in the specialty of pediatric nursing, and has appropriate credentials in the State where they practice as an Advanced Practice Registered Nurse (APRN).[1]

The Advanced Practice Task Force of the Society of Pediatric Nurses (SPN) has undertaken the development of advanced practice standards in response to the need expressed by Advanced Practice Registered Nurses (APRNs) across the nation for published standards to assist in clarifying advanced practice roles to healthcare professionals, including other nurses, administrators, third-party-payers, legislators, and the public.[2] These standards are also necessary as a precursor to the continued development of certification processes for Advanced Practice Pediatric Nurses (APPNs).

A variety of definitions of the APRN have been developed:

> Nurses in advanced clinical nursing practice have a graduate degree and/or certification in nursing. They conduct comprehensive health assessments; demonstrate a high level of autonomy and expert skill in diagnosis and treatment of complex responses of individuals, families, and communities to actual or potential health problems. They formulate clinical decisions to manage acute and chronic illness and promote wellness. Nurses in advanced practice integrate education, research, management, leadership, and consultation into their clinical role and function in collegial relationships with nursing peers, physicians, and others who influence the health environment.[2]

> The advanced practice of nursing means practice based on the knowledge and skills acquired in a nursing education, through licensure as a registered nurse, and a graduate degree with a major in nursing or a graduate degree with a concentration in an advanced nursing practice category, which includes both didactic and clinical components, advanced knowledge in nursing theory, physical and psychosocial assessment, appropriate interventions, and management of health care.[26]

While APRNs can have a variety of roles and employment titles, the classic Advanced Practice Pediatric Nurse titles used over the past three decades include Pediatric Clinical Nurse Specialist (PCNS) and Pediatric Nurse Practitioner (PNP). Specialization in pediatrics can also be noted in clinical nurse specialist and nurse practitioner roles that include pediatrics or a subgroup of pediatric patients in their overall patient practice population. These would include:

- Family Nurse Practitioners and Clinical Nurse Specialists
- Neonatal Nurse Practitioners and Clinical Nurse Specialists
- Developmental Disabilities Clinical Nurse Specialists
- Certified Nurse Midwives (CNMs)
- Certified Registered Nurse Anesthetists (CRNAs)

CNMs and CRNAs are expected to incorporate advanced knowledge of pediatric concepts into their clinical practice because their client populations include pediatric patients and their families. Therefore, advanced practice pediatric nursing could be equally applicable to nurses serving as CNMs or CRNAs or in nurse practitioner or clinical nurse specialist roles that include pediatric patients in their clinical practice population. Historically, APRN roles have been distinct in practice setting, scope of practice, and educational requirements. Today the focus is toward bringing all APRNs, including CNMs and CRNAs, into conceptual unity and recognizing them under the umbrella of advanced practice nursing. This framework does not purport that the practice in each of these roles is similar, but that the common dimensions of practice should be identified and the differences noted to advance the autonomy and authority of advanced practice nurses.

The following descriptions are illustrative of the advanced practice roles that require knowledge specialization and clinical expertise in the care of children and their families. The focus here is on the Clinical Nurse Specialist and the Nurse Practitioner.

Pediatric Clinical Nurse Specialists (PCNS)—The PCNS is an APRN prepared in the clinical nursing specialty of pediatric nursing to provide direct patient care and to serve as a leader in education, research, quality assurance, outcome monitoring, and consultation with other nurses, health team members, and the community. CNSs are prepared at the master's or doctoral level and have demonstrated cost-effective, quality outcomes. PCNSs have demonstrated improved outcomes for children in acute care settings, as well as increasingly in ambulatory, home, and school settings. Previously, CNSs were employed and paid by the institution but many currently work independently, in private or collaborative practice.

Pediatric Nurse Practitioner (PNP)—Pediatric Nurse Practitioners first developed in the late 1960s and gained increased visibility in the 1980s as a result of shortages of physicians to provide primary care in underserved areas of the country. The first PNP program was established in 1965 at the University of Colorado. It was designed to prepare professional nurses to provide comprehensive well-child care as well as to manage common childhood health problems. Project evaluations indicated that PNPs were highly competent in assessing and managing 75% of the health care for well and ill children in the community. The focus of care shifted from managing illness to a strong family-oriented, health promotion focus.

The National Association of Pediatric Nurse Associates and Practitioners (NAPNAP) defines the PNP as a registered nurse who has acquired knowledge and clinical skills in child health through successful completion of a formal education program.[27] PNPs provide primary care including wellness, prevention and health promotion, physical examinations and developmental assessments, and treatment for common childhood illnesses as well as coordination of care for chronic illnesses. PNPs have typically worked in hospital, clinics, or private office settings and can be found working throughout the healthcare continuum. A newer role for Pediatric Nurse Practitioners is that of the pediatric acute care nurse practitioner, working primarily in acute inpatient and critical care settings. These APRNs manage children and adolescents with complex acute and critical health problems.

The total number of APRNs is not known; however, categories of APRNs numbered over 248,000 in 1996 or almost 10% of all RNs. NPs numbered 70,993 and CNSs numbered 53,799. Nurses prepared as APRNs (both NP and CNS) numbered 7,802.[28] About 14.8% (38,471) of all APRNs are specialists in pediatric nursing; about one-half of these are master's prepared. About 10% of all Advanced Practice Pediatric Nurses are from minority groups.[29-30]

APRNs from all specialties have consistently provided increased accessibility to high quality, cost-effective health care for families.[19,21,22,31] As healthcare reform and organizational restructuring have taken place throughout the 1990s, the diverse roles of Advanced Practice Pediatric Nurses have reconfigured expected skills, practice sites, practice focus, and organizational agendas. For instance, Pediatric Clinical Nurse Specialist practice has evolved to increasingly emphasize physical assessment and clinical decision making.

The PNP role has increasingly emphasized more leadership activities. Thus, all APRNs now work within a "larger" healthcare system and need to be current and competent in direct patient care, and comfortable serving as change agents and leaders in their practice setting.

Advanced Practice Pediatric Nurses have increasingly been used to meet a variety of diversified roles that are evolving from those traditionally provided by master's prepared pediatric nurses. Roles in primary care still flourish. The acute care and critical care APPN has also demonstrated effectiveness in managing the needs of children in the inpatient setting. Additionally, collaborative practice with other providers and among advanced practice nurses has used the strengths of each role to provide complementary services.[32] Community nursing centers, private practices, collaborative practices with physicians, and school-based clinics also have evolved as effective practice arenas for APPNs. The dramatic and dynamic changes and expectations of the APPN's role challenge the traditional thinking of educators, administrators, policy makers, other healthcare providers, and the APPNs themselves. In order for APPNs to meet the needs of children and their families, the profession must work to optimize the clinical, education, regulatory, and certification environments.

Key Elements and Defining Characteristics of the Advanced Practice Nurse

The key elements and defining characteristics that delineate the uniqueness of all APRNs include the components of educational background, clinical practice focus, and role dimensions. Table 2 summarizes these key elements and characteristics as they apply to the Advanced Practice Pediatric Nurse.

Table 2: *Defining Characteristics of Advanced Practice Pediatric Nurses.*[1,31]

Key Elements	Defining Characteristics
Educational background	Graduate or doctoral education in the APRN role, and clinical specialization in pediatric nursing
	Certification in the role and clinical specialty of Advanced Practice Pediatric Nursing
Clinical practice focus	Expertise in clinical practice (expanded nursing and medical procedures) with children and their families • Comprehensive health assessment, including growth and development • Diagnosis and treatment (including prescriptive treatment) of complex responses to actual or potential health problems of children within the context of their families and communities • Management of acute or chronic illnesses, and promotion and maintenance of wellness • Management of restorative and rehabilitative practices to enhance the quality of life for children and their families
Role dimensions	Integration of education, research, management, leadership, and consultation into clinical role
	Change agent skills
	Ethical decision-making skills related to pediatric issues and dilemmas
	Autonomy of practice
	Design, direction, implementation, and evaluation of programs to serve at-risk pediatric populations in the community

The scope of practice of the Advanced Practice Pediatric Nurse builds upon knowledge and experience in pediatric nursing, plus the expanded knowledge, skills, and expertise of advanced education. The ANA has described the APRN role to include specialization, expansion of practice skills, and advancement (graduate education). Specialization involves focus on one specific area of nursing: pediatric nursing. Expansion involves additional skills and knowledge in pediatric clinical practice, including nursing and some medical practice skills. Advancement combines both specialization and expansion through in-depth study of the research-based, theoretical, and clinical practice issues unique to the pediatric population. APRNs may overlap with some of the diagnostic and treatment skills historically found in medical practice. The APRN is a professional nurse with expanded skills, knowledge, and expertise in pediatric advanced practice nursing.[33]

Impediments to the full use of advanced practice nurses include: 1) legal barriers such as laws that require physician supervision or limit a nurse's prescriptive authority, 2) financial barriers that prevent public and private payers from reimbursing advanced practice nurses, and 3) professional barriers.[34] Safriet[22] stated "Advanced practice nurses have demonstrated repeatedly that they can provide cost-effective, high quality primary care for many of the neediest members of society, but their role has been severely limited by restrictions on their scope of practice, prescriptive authority, and eligibility for reimbursement" (p. 417).

Settings for Pediatric Nursing Practice

Inpatient Setting

The inpatient setting provides one of the richest and most diverse arenas for implementing the role of child healthcare provider. To date, there exist 81 hospitals or medical centers in the United States and 4 in Canada whose sole focus is on providing acute care or rehabilitation services to the pediatric population. Thousands of additional facilities exist in which pediatric specialty areas (e.g., pediatric units, pediatric intensive care, adolescent units, neonatal intensive care units) are services provided within the multi-focused acute care setting. In addition, because of the changes brought on by managed care and healthcare reform, nurses in all acute care arenas will likely have contact with pediatric clients sometime over the course of their nursing practice.

Outpatient Clinics and Offices

For most children and their families, the singular access to, and ongoing contact with, healthcare professionals will be through a clinic or a physician's office. Through ongoing contact with the family, the nurse in this setting has an opportunity to develop a mutually gratifying and therapeutic relationship with the family. The evolving exposure to the well or chronically ill child allows the clinic or office nurse and the Advanced Practice Pediatric Nurse to have a more complete picture of the child's general well-being and ability to achieve developmental milestones. Illness prevention and health promotion activities are the core interventions of the nurse and the healthcare team. For children coping with a chronic illness, the health care team may also focus on maintaining optimum levels of health.

The clinic or office provides an ideal setting to provide health teaching to the child and the caregiver. Several studies have attempted to quantify the amount of time spent by health professionals providing counseling and health teaching during clinic visits. Despite the fact that parents view health teaching as one of their greatest needs, the time spent in this activity is embarrassingly short. One classic study of pediatricians indicated that the average time for a well-child visit was 10 minutes, with 90 seconds of that time devoted to providing anticipatory health teaching.[35] In even the busiest clinics, the health team can use a variety of carefully selected educational media to launch discussions regarding normal developmental milestones, identification and treatment of common childhood illnesses, and therapy regimes applicable to the child's diagnosis. Videos, pamphlets, coloring books, toys, and the Internet are educational tools the clinic or office nurse can use to augment face-to-face discussions with the child and family.

The clinic or office nurse may also be called upon to participate in research projects directed and approved by the managing healthcare team. Most importantly, the ongoing relationship the nurse has established with the child may help identify any unwarranted side effects of a research protocol.

The nurse working in a specialty pediatric clinic collaborates with a multidisciplinary team to meet the challenges of patients with a chronic or terminal illness. Visits to the clinic by these children often require great coordination to ensure that all disciplines who need to see the child are able to do so, to ensure that the family's valuable time is not wasted, and to ascertain that ongoing well child care is being addressed. The nurse serves as a vital link in the communication process between health team members and the family.

Community Health Care

Within the domain of community health, child healthcare issues are a dominant area of concern. The nurse with skills and knowledge in child health care can contribute in immeasurable ways to the many child health programs initiated by community health organizations. These programs include efforts aimed at decreasing infant mortality and increasing prenatal care, decreasing the incidence of accidental injuries among children, preventing lead poisoning, providing immunization programs, decreasing the incidence of child abuse and neglect, and eliminating adolescent substance use.[36] It has been said that child health status is an important indicator of the health of the nation. Keeping this statement in mind, the nurse with a strong affiliation toward children's health issues has the opportunity to positively affect large populations of children and their families through the role of a community health practitioner.

Home Health Care

Though home care practices have been shaped by roots in community nursing practice, home care nurses work primarily with ill individuals and their families. Home care requires that the nurse address the environmental, social, and personal factors affecting health, as does community health nursing practice. The emphasis in home care, however, is upon working with individuals rather than with population groups. Generally, home care is appropriate whenever a person needs assistance that cannot be easily or effectively provided by family members or friends on an ongoing basis.[37]

Children are referred to a home care agency based on their diagnosis or disease, their need for treatment of a condition, or for assistance in working through the end stages of a terminal disease. The focus is on preventing admission to an acute care setting, providing assistance to families, and giving direct treatment in the home.[38] The environmental, social, psychological, and economic impact on the patient is assessed and included in the treatment plan. In addition, it cannot be forgotten that the family's home is their domain. Parents play the central role in implementation of care for the child. Family goals and preferences take priority in the home care plan.[11] The need for collaborative practice is critical.

School Settings

Nurses have become established and required associates of the faculty in both private and public schools. Today's school nurse may be employed by a local school system, or by a county, city, or state governmental agency. The school nurse is required to have obtained a bachelor's degree in nursing and continuing education hours specializing in the role and services of the school nurse.

At one time, a model existed in which a nurse was located at most school sites. Today, with budget cuts presenting continuing challenges to school districts, the school nurse is often found trying to meet the needs of several schools. In these cases, a nurse's aide or a health clerk may be responsible for monitoring minor day-to-day health problems at a school. The nurse is responsible for overall management and delegation of activities to the aides and for evaluating the appropriateness of interventions provided to ailing children.

The newest approach to providing comprehensive health care to young people, especially those from low-income families, is school-based health centers, also referred to as school-based clinics. These clinics are located inside the school grounds and are not the same as school-linked clinics, which are off-site and thus not as accessible to the students on a day-to-day basis. School-based clinics try to capitalize on many features associated with easy access— convenience, comfort, confidentiality, and cost. The school-based clinic can address these health concerns and provide health education to students of all ages.

In general, staffing within school-based clinics includes a pediatric nurse practitioner or physician's assistant, a clinic assistant or receptionist, and an assortment of health educators, physicians, nutritionists, nurses, and social workers. These staff are trained to deal with the unique growth, social, developmental, and emotional needs of the school-age population they serve. Activities of the clinic may include once-a-year health fairs, ongoing participation in crisis intervention teams, in-class health education, parent education, teacher training, sports medicine clinics, student health clubs, question-and-answer columns in student newspapers, sponsoring immunization programs, involvement in dropout prevention initiatives, and assessing health risk behaviors of their populations.[39-40] Pediatric nurses, nurse practitioners, and public health nurses are the backbone of these clinics, providing the specialty nurse with a rich and diverse clinical setting in which to develop a rewarding career.

Air and Surface Transport Nursing

The first helicopter transport of a premature infant occurred in 1967. The 3-pound, 7-ounce baby survived the 202-mile flight from Zion, Illinois, but died three days later due to congenital abnormalities. With no research literature to consult, these early pediatric and neonatal flight teams had to discover new ways to contend with the effects of altitude, temperature, motion, airplane noise, and other factors on the sick child. From the growing emphasis on pediatric transport, a Pediatric Special Interest Group has been formed within the Air and Surface Transport Nurses Association (ASTNA), formerly known as the National Flight Nurses Association (NFNA). Approximately 40 to 50% of pediatric air transports involve children less than 1 year of age, with 20 to 30% of the children 1 to 3 years of age.

Many of the infants using air or surface transport systems are technologically dependent and are being transferred from community hospitals to a Level III Neonatal Intensive Care Unit to have their acute care needs better met. Generally young children and adolescents are transported to a Pediatric Intensive Care Unit or a Step-Down Unit from a community site. Most pediatric and neonatal air and surface ambulance programs today are sponsored by single hospitals. Hospital consortia, public agencies (such as the Highway

Patrol), and a handful of freestanding companies only account for about 5% of the programs nationwide.[41]

The transport team responding to a pediatric health crisis must possess a variety of specialized skills and abilities. Pediatric specialty teams are typically composed of an RN/RN, RN/MD or RN/MD/Respiratory Therapist team. Certification is available for the flight nurse. Completion of pediatric advanced life support (PALS) and a neonatal resuscitation program (NRP) is required for transport team members in most programs.[42-43]

Camp Settings

For the pediatric nurse who enjoys the challenges of the wilderness, camp nursing can be an exciting respite from other full-time professional responsibilities. A camp nurse is responsible for all aspects of health care in a camp setting. Most camps encourage experienced pediatric nurses (two years or more) to apply. Applicants should have Basic Life Support training and Basic First Aid Training and must function within their scope of nursing practice.[44] However, student nurses and nursing faculty can also benefit from the camp nurse experience. Students who serve as counselors or nurse assistants can learn more about normal child growth and development as well as practice technical nursing skills. Clinical placements at specialty camps for the chronically ill offer the student an opportunity to better understand the impact of the illness upon the child and the family. Faculty have an opportunity to maintain and upgrade their clinical expertise in a unique setting far from the hospital corridors. The camp community also offers an accessible population for nursing research studies.

In addition to the generalized camp setting, there are specialty camps for children with chronic or terminal illnesses, such as those for children with cancer, cystic fibrosis, asthma, and developmental disabilities. Health facilities at specialty camps permit children in treatment to continue their health care. Because all the children attending the camp are in some phase of a treatment or a remission cycle, seeing other children undergo various therapies for their condition is not an unusual or unsettling sight. Through the camp experience the children can informally share their concerns or fears with their new-found friends, or with counselors specially trained to understand the needs of chronically and terminally ill children.

The primary goal of the specialty camps is to allow the children, who may have had extensive or unpleasant medical treatment and life experiences, to enjoy a real camping experience. The camp programs do not intend to change the child's usual routines or diets, therapies or resting periods; rather, the child's unique needs are accommodated to enable the child to enjoy the experience and leave with pleasant memories.[45] Nursing care is available 24 hours a day, with visits and treatments provided in the child's cabin, if requested.

Education

Education guidelines for the generalist level of pediatric nursing have been outlined in the *Standards and Guidelines for Pre-licensure and Professional Education for the Nursing Care of Children and Their Families.*[6-7] This document was published in 1995 with the intent of providing a new vision of education to prepare pre-licensure students and new graduates for the complex care of children and their families.[6-7,46-47] The standards contain 11 concepts in 3 domains of knowledge and skills that should be included in every educational program preparing nurses. The document does not produce the curriculum that should be provided within one specific course or set of courses about child health care. Rather, the standards state the goals, process criteria, and outcome criteria for the 11 concepts that can be integrated into all content areas and clinical settings where the needs of children and their families should be discussed. As a collaborator in developing this document, the Society of Pediatric Nurses strongly believes this document will serve as a guiding force to direct nursing education for the care of children in our complex society.

Educational guidelines for Advanced Practice Pediatric Nursing are outlined in the appendix of this document. They are consistent with other national educational standards. In 1996, the American Association of Colleges of Nursing (AACN) outlined a master's in nursing curriculum which detailed a generic core content for all students, including research, policy, organization and financing of health care, ethics, professional role development, theoretical foundations of nursing practice, human diversity and social issues, and health promotion and disease prevention. A specialty core curriculum for APRNs who provide direct clinical care included advanced health and physical assessment, advanced pathophysiology, and advanced pharmacology. Likewise the National Organization of Nurse Practitioner Faculties[48] has developed curriculum guidelines for nurse practitioners, incorporating the full scope of advanced practice nursing. The American College of Nurse-Midwives[49] has established accreditation criteria for educational programs and the American Association of Nurse Anesthetists[50] has created accreditation standards for nurse anesthetist educational programs. These guidelines and standards apply to graduate education and emphasize direct care across settings.

Education of Advanced Practice Pediatric Nurses includes specialty content in advanced health and physical assessment of the child, advanced pathophysiology, advanced pharmacology for children, advanced growth and development, family theory, promotion and maintenance of optimal health for children and families, and management of acute and chronic conditions in children.[51-52] Faculty and preceptors for Advanced Practice Pediatric Nurses need expertise in research or clinical practice, and experience in a variety of conditions and settings where children receive health care.

Certification

Certification is a process in which a voluntary, governing agency validates a registered nurse's qualifications, knowledge, and scope of practice in a defined clinical or functional area of nursing.[53] A nurse becomes certified upon meeting eligibility requirements of the certifying agency and upon passing a written examination that tests the nurse's knowledge of current practice standards in a selected area of nursing. Through this process the agency or professional organization acknowledges for the individual and to the general public that the individual has mastered a body of knowledge for a particular specialty.[54] There are currently 28 nursing organizations in the United States that provide certification services. For the pediatric nurse the primary agencies providing certification in this specialty area include the American Nurses Credentialing Center; the Certification Corporation of Pediatric Oncology Nurses; the National

Certification Board of Pediatric Nurse Practitioners and Nurses; and the National Certification Corporation for the Obstetric, Gynecologic and Neonatal Nurse Specialties.

Professional certification is required to practice as a nurse practitioner in 31 states and as a clinical nurse specialist in 18 states with the number of states requiring certification increasing for both. Professional certification to measure clinical competence for Advanced Practice Pediatric Nurses is provided for the CNS or PNP through the American Nurses Credentialing Center (ANCC) or for the PNP by the National Certification Board of Pediatric Nurse Practitioners and Nurses (NCBPNP/N). These certification examinations focus on primary care. A new certification examination provided by the NCBPNP/N will certify pediatric acute care nurse practitioners.

Many specialty nursing organizations offer certification in their respective specialties, which may or may not include a differentiated examination for Advanced Practice Pediatric Nurses. For instance, the American Association of Critical Care Nurses now offers certification for Critical Care Pediatric Clinical Nurse Specialists and the Oncology Nursing Society offers certification for Advanced Practice Pediatric Oncology Nurses.

Regulation

State Nurse Practice Acts provide direction for the regulation of all nurses, including advanced practice of nurses in the state. State APRN statutes vary widely from title protection to specific delineation of APRN practice. The autonomy of practice ranges from private practice with referral options to practicing under the supervision of a physician. In 1993, the National Council of State Boards of Nursing (NCSBN) approved a position statement in support of second licensure for advanced practice.[26] The position of the ANA on this subject consistently supports one scope of nursing practice, one licensure for registered nurses, and minimal statutory language about advanced practice. The ANA proposes that state constituent member associations promote specific designations of APRN roles in rules and regulations instead of law to avoid attaching statutory language to the roles. Additionally, the profession is to develop consistent standards of regulation through certification, peer review, and continuing education to self-regulate the role so that the profession retains the responsibility and accountability for regulating practice.[1]

STANDARDS OF PEDIATRIC NURSING PRACTICE

Definition and Role of Standards

Standards are authoritative statements in which the nursing profession describes the responsibilities for which its practitioners are accountable to the public and the client outcomes for which nurses are responsible. Consequently, standards reflect the values and priorities of the profession. Standards provide direction for professional nursing practice and a framework for the evaluation of practice. Written in measurable terms, standards also define the nursing profession's accountability to the public and the client outcomes for which nurses are responsible.

Development of Standards

Standards of professional nursing practice may pertain to general or specialty practice. A professional nursing organization has a responsibility to its membership and the public it serves to develop standards of practice. As a professional specialty organization for pediatric nurses, the Society of Pediatric Nurses (SPN) has developed specialty standards that apply to the practice of professional nurses who care for children and their families.

This publication sets forth standards of pediatric nursing practice and applies them to all nurses engaged in the care of children and their families across care settings. It is based on the *Statement on the Scope and Standards of Pediatric Clinical Nursing Practice*,[51] the *Standards of Clinical Nursing Practice*,[56] and the *Scope and Standards of Advanced Practice Registered Nursing*.[1] The *Scope and Standards of Pediatric Nursing Practice* describes a competent level of professional nursing care and professional performance common to nurses engaged in the care of children and their families based on their generalist or advanced practice roles.

Assumptions

Scope and Standards of Pediatric Nursing Practice focuses primarily on the processes of providing pediatric nursing care and performing professional role activities. These standards apply to all nurses involved in the care of children and their families despite the tremendous variability in environments in which nurses practice. Recognizing the link between the professional work environment and the nurse's ability to deliver care, employers must provide an environment supportive of nursing practice.

A second assumption is that nursing care is individualized to meet a particular child's or family's unique needs and situation. This includes respect for the child's and family's goals and preferences in developing and implementing a plan of care. Given that one of the nurse's primary responsibilities is patient education, nurses provide children and their families with adequate information to make informed decisions and to attain assent or informed permission regarding their health care and treatment, including health promotion, prevention of disease, and attainment of a peaceful death.

The third assumption is that the nurse establishes a partnership with the child, family, and other healthcare providers. In this partnership, the nurse works collaboratively to coordinate care provided to the child and the family. The degree of participation by the child and family will vary based upon preference and ability, and in the case of the child, upon age, developmental abilities, and cognitive understanding of the plan of care.

Organizing Principles of the Scope and Standards of Pediatric Nursing Practice

According to *Nursing's Social Policy Statement*," the recipients of nursing care are individuals, groups, families, or communities...The recipient(s) of nursing care can be referred to as patient(s), client(s), or person(s)."[3] The Scope and Standards of Pediatric Nursing Practice uses the terms "patient," "child," and "family" to indicate the person(s) to whom the nurse is providing services as sanctioned by the state Nurse Practice Act. Care can be provided to assist the child or family, sick or well, in performance of those activities contributing to health or its recovery (or to peaceful death) that the child or family would perform unaided if the child or family had the necessary strength, will, or knowledge, and to do this in such a way as to help the child or family gain independence as rapidly as possible. The cultural, racial, developmental, and ethnic diversity of the child and the family must always be taken into account in providing nursing services.

The *Scope and Standards of Pediatric Nursing Practice* applies to all registered nurses engaged in the nursing care of children and their families, regardless of clinical specialty, practice setting, or educational preparation. Standards that further define the responsibilities of nurses working with children and families in advanced practice roles are articulated in this document. Nurses practicing at an advanced level of practice will be accountable for meeting the standards of pediatric nursing practice, as well as the scope and standards for advanced practice pediatric nursing outlined in this document and in the *Scope and Standards of Advanced Practice Registered Nursing.*[1]

The *Scope and Standards of Pediatric Nursing Practice* consists of "Standards of Care" and "Standards of Professional Performance," which include the following:

Standards of Care

- Assessment
- Diagnosis
- Outcome Identification
- Planning
- Implementation
  - Case Management
  - Consultation
  - Health Promotion, Health Maintenance, and Health Teaching
  - Prescriptive Authority
  - Referral
- Evaluation

Standards of Professional Performance

- Quality of Care
- Performance Appraisal
- Education
- Collegiality
- Ethics
- Collaboration
- Research
- Resource Utilization

Standards of Care

The six standards of care describe a competent level of nursing care, as demonstrated by the nursing process, including assessment, diagnosis, outcome identification, planning, implementation, and evaluation. The nursing process encompasses all significant actions taken by nurses in providing care to all patients and family, and forms the foundation of clinical decision making. Several themes cut across all areas of nursing practice and reflect nursing responsibilities for all children and their families. These themes merit additional attention, and include:

- Providing age-appropriate and culturally and ethnically sensitive care
- Maintaining a safe environment
- Educating children and their families about health practices and treatment modalities
- Providing care that is family-centered
- Ensuring continuity of care
- Coordinating care across settings and among caregivers
- Managing information
- Communicating effectively

These themes will be reflected in the measurement criteria associated with various standards in this document, although the wording may be different. They are highlighted here because they are fundamental to many of the standards, and because they have emerged as being consistently and significantly influential in nursing practice today. With the next revision of this document, some of these themes will undoubtedly evolve into standard statements in and of themselves.

Standards of Professional Performance

The eight standards of professional performance describe a competent level of behavior in the professional role—including activities related to quality of care, performance appraisal, education, collegiality, ethics, collaboration, research, and resource utilization. Within these standards the advanced practice nurse is expected to be accountable for several other responsibilities that comprise the hallmarks of the profession and of the advanced practice role. These activities include serving in leadership positions within a professional organization, serving as a role model or mentor to other pediatric nurses, and participating in the conduct of family-centered research. All nurses are expected to engage in professional role activities appropriate to their education, position, and practice setting. Ultimately, nurses are accountable to themselves, patients, and peers for their professional actions.

Criteria

Criteria are key indicators of competent practice. *Scope and Standards of Pediatric Nursing Practice* includes criteria that allow the standards to be measured. These criteria include key indicators of competent practice. For the standards to be met, all criteria must be met, with additional criteria requirements for the advanced practice nurse. Standards should remain stable over time, as they reflect the philosophical values of the profession. However, criteria can be revised to incorporate advancements in scientific knowledge and clinical practice. Criteria must remain consistent with current nursing practice and research.

Throughout this document, terms such as "appropriate," "pertinent," and "realistic" are used. A document like this cannot account for all possible scenarios that the pediatric nurse might encounter in clinical practice. The pediatric nurse will need to exercise judgment based on education and experience in determining what is appropriate, pertinent, or realistic. Further direction may be available from documents such as guidelines for practice or agency standards, policies, procedures, and protocols.

Guidelines

Guidelines describe a process of patient care management which has the potential for improving the quality of clinical and consumer decision-making. As systematically developed statements based on available scientific evidence and expert opinion, guidelines address the care of specific patient populations or phenomena, whereas standards provide a broad framework for practice. Many practice guidelines have been developed by professional organizations that are applicable to the pediatric population. Such guidelines should be used to provide direction for clinical practice policies, procedures, and protocols.

Summary

Scope and Standards of Pediatric Nursing Practice delineates the professional responsibilities of registered nurses engaged in clinical practice related to children and their families, regardless of setting. *Scope and Standards of Pediatric Nursing Practice* and nursing practice guidelines could serve as a basis for:

- Quality improvement systems
- Data bases
- Regulatory systems
- Healthcare reimbursement and financing methodologies
- Development and evaluation of nursing service delivery systems and organizational structures
- Certification activities
- Job descriptions and performance appraisals
- Agency policies, procedures, and protocols
- Educational offerings
- Research activities
- Consistency in care

In order to best serve the public and the nursing profession, nursing must continue to develop standards of practice and practice guidelines. Nursing must examine how standards and practice guidelines can be disseminated and used more effectively to enhance and promote the quality of clinical practice. In addition, standards and practice guidelines must be evaluated on an ongoing basis, with revisions made as necessary. The dynamic nature of the healthcare environment and the growing body of nursing research provide both the impetus and the opportunity for nursing to ensure competent clinical practice and to promote ongoing professional development and client care.

STANDARDS OF CARE

Comprehensive pediatric nursing care focuses on helping children and their families and communities achieve their optimum health potentials. This is best achieved within the framework of family-centered care and the pediatric nursing process including primary, secondary, and tertiary care coordinated across health care and community settings.

Standard 1. Assessment

The pediatric nurse collects patient health data.

Measurement Criteria

1. Data collection involves the child, family, other individuals important to the family, and other healthcare providers as appropriate.

2. The priority of data collection activities is determined by the child's immediate condition or needs.

3. Pertinent data are collected using appropriate assessment techniques and instruments specific for the child's age.

    *   The physical assessment may include but be not limited to:
        *   Height and weight (current and pre-illness)
        *   Vital signs
        *   Nutritional status (anthropometrics)
        *   Physical examination
        *   Head circumference (age-appropriate)

    *   Behavioral assessment may include but not be limited to:
        *   Affect and activity
        *   Interactions, appropriate for age, with adults and peers
        *   Behavioral differences across settings (home, school, clinic, hospital)

    *   Developmental assessment may include but not be limited to:
        *   Personal and social
        *   Language

- Fine motor and adaptive
- Gross motor
- Cognitive
- Emotional and mental health

- Family assessment may include but not be limited to:
  - Familial strengths
  - Cultural background
  - Racial background
  - Ethnic background
  - Socioeconomic background
  - Religious or spiritual background
  - Coping strategies
  - Learning style
  - Injury prevention and safety practices
  - Preferences of family for receiving information and support
  - Ways the family would like to be involved in the child's health care

4. Data collection should include health history when appropriate. The nurse should collect data in ways that convey respect for families. A health history may include but is not limited to:

- Birth history (age-appropriate)
- Growth and development milestones
- Past medical illness or surgeries
- Family history, including genetic history and congenital abnormalities, mental retardation, metabolic problems, and mental illness
- Accidents or injuries
- Educational needs related to maximizing the child's health
- Behavioral patterns and individual strengths
- Communicable or childhood diseases
- Exposure to hazardous agents
- Dietary habits and intake history
- Growth parameters as compared with normal for age
- Significant trends in weight gain or loss
- Immunization status
- Sexual history (age-appropriate)
- Substance abuse history (age-appropriate)

- Experience with pain and pain management techniques
- School history (age-appropriate)
- Elimination patterns
- Sleep patterns and sleep aids
- Information that family members see as significant
- Family observations of the child
- Strengths of the child and family
- Any significant stress; comforting and coping strategies
- Relationships with the family, including the potential for abuse
- Socioeconomic, cultural, spiritual, and environmental factors
- Peer relationships

5. Relevant data are synthesized, prioritized, and documented in a retrievable form.

6. The data collection process is systematic and ongoing.

Additional Measurement Criteria for the Advanced Practice Pediatric Nurse

7. Assessment techniques are based on research and knowledge.

8. Data collected is based on clinical judgment to ensure relevant and necessary data are collected about the child, the family, and the community of influence.

9. Diagnostic tests and procedures relevant to the child's current status are initiated as indicated and are interpreted.

Standard 2. Diagnosis

The pediatric nurse analyzes the assessment data in determining diagnoses.

Measurement Criteria

1. Diagnoses and risk factors are derived from the assessment data.

2. Diagnoses are discussed, validated, and prioritized with the child, family, significant others, and other healthcare providers when possible and appropriate.

3. Diagnoses are developmentally appropriate, age-appropriate, and culturally sensitive.

4. Diagnoses include those that are specific to areas of growth, development, and family dynamics.

5. Diagnoses are documented in a manner that facilitates the determination of expected outcomes and plan of care.

Additional Measurement Criteria for the Advanced Practice Pediatric Nurse

6. Diagnoses, nursing or selected medical, are derived from analysis of the assessment data using appropriate complex clinical reasoning.

7. Diagnoses related to disease and injury prevention, health promotion, restoration, and maintenance are determined.

8. A differential diagnosis is formulated by systematically comparing and contrasting clinical findings.

9. Diagnoses are made using advanced synthesis of information obtained during the interview with the child and the family, the physical examination of the child, and diagnostic tests or procedures performed on the child.

10. Diagnoses are continually evaluated and revised as appropriate to ongoing assessment data.

11. Diagnoses conform to an accepted classification system (as defined by the healthcare setting) and are documented in a manner that facilitates determination of expected outcomes and plan of care.

Standard 3. Outcome Identification

The pediatric nurse identifies expected outcomes individualized to the child and the family.

Measurement Criteria

1. Outcomes are derived from the diagnoses.

2. Outcomes are mutually formulated with the child (age-appropriate), family, and other healthcare providers when possible and appropriate.

3. Outcomes are developmentally appropriate, age-appropriate, and culturally sensitive.

4. Outcomes are family-centered.

5. Outcomes are realistic in relation to the child's and family's potential capabilities.

6. Outcomes are attainable in relation to resources available to the child and family.

7. Outcomes include a time estimate for attainment and are prioritized as appropriate.

8. Outcomes provide direction for continuity of care.

9. Outcomes are documented as measurable goals.

Additional Measurement Criteria for the Advanced Practice Pediatric Nurse

10. Expected outcomes are identified with consideration of the associated risks, benefits, and costs for the child and family.

11. Expected outcomes are consistent with current scientific and clinical practice knowledge.

12. Expected outcomes are modified based on changes in the child's condition.

13. Expected outcomes provide direction for continuity of care for the child and family.

14. Expected outcomes serve as a record of change in the child's health status.

Standard 4. Planning

The pediatric nurse develops a plan of care that prescribes interventions to attain expected outcomes.

Measurement Criteria

1. The plan is individualized to the child's condition and the child's and family's needs.

2. The plan is developed with the child (age appropriate), family, and other healthcare providers, as appropriate.

3. The plan reflects current pediatric nursing practice.

4. The plan provides for continuity of care.

5. The plan is family-centered.

6. The plan is developmentally appropriate, age-appropriate, and culturally sensitive.

7. The plan includes areas specific to growth and development.

8. The plan is dynamic and flexible and reassessed as needed.

9. Priorities for care are established.

10. The plan is documented.

Additional Measurement Criteria for the Advanced Practice Pediatric Nurse

11. The comprehensive plan of care describes the diverse assessment and diagnostic strategies and the therapeutic interventions that reflect current pediatric healthcare knowledge, research, and practice.

12. The comprehensive plan of care reflects the responsibilities of the advanced practice pediatric nurse, and the patient and family and may include delegation of responsibilities and consultation to assist others in implementing the plan of care.

13. The comprehensive plan of care addresses strategies for promotion and restoration of health and prevention of illness, injury, and disease through independent clinical decision-making.

14. The comprehensive plan of care includes educational interventions related to the child's health status, therapies, and self-care activities.

15. The comprehensive plan of care provides for appropriate referrals and coordination of comprehensive services to ensure continuity of care.

16. The comprehensive plan of care is documented in a manner that allows access by the child, the family, and healthcare providers as appropriate and provides direction for the family and the healthcare team as they focus on attaining expected outcomes.

Standard 5. Implementation

The pediatric nurse implements the interventions identified in the plan of care.

Measurement Criteria

1. Interventions are consistent with the established plan of care.

2. Interventions are implemented in a safe, timely, and appropriate manner.

3. Interventions are family-centered.

4. Interventions are developmentally appropriate, age-appropriate, and culturally sensitive.

5. Interventions include meeting the growth and development needs of the child and the family.

6. Interventions are individualized to the child's condition and the child's and family's needs.

7. Children of accountable age and ability are encouraged in self-responsibility related to care.

8. Interventions include anticipatory guidance, information about injury and disease prevention, and home care management as appropriate for the child's developmental level, provided to the child or the caregiver.

9. Interventions are documented.

*Additional Measurement Criteria for the Advanced Practice
Pediatric Nurse*

10. Interventions and treatments are performed or implemented with knowledge of pediatric healthcare research findings and reflect a scientific basis and theory.

11. Interventions and treatments are performed within the scope of advanced practice registered nursing and according to appropriate regulatory statutes.

12. Interventions and treatments are performed after the Advanced Practice Pediatric Nurse has received appropriate education or training and has demonstrated proficiency in the skill or procedure being employed.

5a. Case Management and Coordination of Comprehensive Health Services

The Advanced Practice Pediatric Nurse works with the family to coordinate the child's healthcare services across settings to achieve optimal quality of care, delivered in a cost-effective manner within an interdisciplinary team approach.

Measurement Criteria

1. Appropriate monitoring, assessments, and interventions are delegated according to the condition of the child and the relative skill and scope of practice of the caregiver.

2. Case management and clinical coordination of care are provided using sophisticated data synthesis with consideration of the child and family's complex needs and desired outcomes. This results in integration of health care that is accessible, available, high quality, and cost effective.

3. Health-related services and additional specialized care are negotiated with the child, the family, appropriate systems, agencies, and providers.

5b. Consultation

The Advanced Practice Pediatric Nurse provides consultation to healthcare providers and others to influence the plan of care for children, to enhance the abilities of others to provide health care, and to effect change in the system.

Measurement Criteria

1. Consultation activities are based on theoretical frameworks, including those that focus on family systems and family-centered care.

2. Consultation is based on mutual respect, and role responsibility is established with the child, the family, and other primary caregivers.

3. Consultation is initiated through mutual identification of the needs for intervention and problem identification.

4. Consultation recommendations are communicated in terms that facilitate understanding and involve the child and the family in decision making.

5. The decision to implement the system change or plan of care remains the responsibility of the child and the family.

6. Mechanisms to implement the interdisciplinary plan of care for the child are initiated by the Advanced Practice Pediatric Nurse with consideration given to the child's unique developmental needs and abilities and the family's level of adaptation and ability to cope with the child's health concerns.

5c. Health Promotion, Restoration, Health Maintenance, and Health Teaching

The Advanced Practice Pediatric Nurse employs diverse and complex strategies, interventions, and teaching with the child and the family to promote, maintain, restore, and improve health, and to prevent illness and injury.

Measurement Criteria

1. Health promotion and disease, illness, and injury prevention strategies include anticipatory guidance and teaching based on current scientific knowledge, research, epidemiological principles, and the family's health beliefs and practices.

2. Health promotion, maintenance, restoration, and teaching methods are appropriate to the culture, age, and developmental cognitive levels for learning needs, readiness to learn, and ability to learn.

3. Appropriate information about potential benefits, risks, complications, and alternatives is provided to the child and family regarding the intervention.

5d. Prescriptive Authority

The Advanced Practice Pediatric Nurse uses prescriptive authority for the purpose of treating symptoms of illness, health promotion, maintenance, or restoration.

Measurement Criteria

1. Treatment interventions and procedures are prescribed in accordance with the child's healthcare needs and based on current pediatric knowledge, research, and practice.

2. Procedures are used and performed as needed in the delivery of comprehensive care to the child.

3. Pharmacological agents are prescribed based on knowledge of pharmacological and physiological principles that are both universal and unique to the care of children at each stage in their developmental life cycle.

4. Specific pharmacological agents or treatments are prescribed based on clinical indicators of the child's status, including but not limited to the results of diagnostic and laboratory tests as appropriate.

5. Intended effects and potential adverse effects of pharmacologic and non-pharmacologic treatments are monitored, and information is provided to the family regarding agents the child should refrain from taking because of the potential adverse effects on the child.

6. Appropriate information about intended effects, potential side effects of the proposed prescription, costs, and alternative treatments and procedures are provided to the child (as appropriate) and family.

7. The Advanced Practice Pediatric Nurse monitors the child's immunization status and, when appropriate, prescribes immunizations to ensure the child is up to date.

5e. Referral

The Advanced Practice Pediatric Nurse identifies the need for additional care and makes referrals as needed.

Measurement Criteria

1. Referrals are discussed with the child (as appropriate) and family.

2. Referrals are made to other healthcare providers and community service agencies as appropriate to the needs of the child with consideration of benefits and costs.

3. As the primary provider, the Advanced Practice Pediatric Nurse ensures continuity of care throughout the healthcare referral process by implementing recommendations from referral sources.

Standard 6. Evaluation

The pediatric nurse evaluates the child's and family's progress toward attainment of outcomes.

Measurement Criteria

1. Evaluation is systematic, ongoing, and criterion-based.

2. The child, family, and other healthcare providers are involved in the evaluation process as appropriate.

3. Ongoing assessment data are used to revise diagnoses, outcomes, and the plan of care as needed.

4. Revisions in diagnoses, outcomes, and the plan of care are documented.

5. The effectiveness of interventions is evaluated in relation to outcomes.

6. The child's and family's readiness for and responses to interventions are documented.

Additional Measurement Criteria for the Advanced Practice Pediatric Nurse

7. The accuracy of diagnoses and effectiveness of interventions are evaluated in relation to the child's attainment of the expected outcomes.

8. The evaluation process is based on advanced knowledge, practice, and research about child health care, and results in revision or resolution of diagnoses, expected outcomes, and plan of care.

STANDARDS OF PROFESSIONAL PERFORMANCE

Standard 1. Quality of Care

The pediatric nurse systematically evaluates the quality and effectiveness of pediatric nursing practice.

Measurement Criteria

1. The pediatric nurse participates in quality-of-care activities as appropriate to that nurse's position, education, and practice environment. Such activities include:

    - Identification of aspects of care important for quality monitoring
    - Analysis of quality data to identify opportunities for improving care
    - Development of policies, procedures, and practice guidelines to improve quality of care, involving families when appropriate
    - Identification of indicators used to monitor quality and effectiveness of nursing care
    - Collection of data to monitor quality and effectiveness of pediatric nursing care, including data from the child and family when appropriate
    - Formulation of recommendations to improve pediatric nursing practice or child and family outcomes
    - Implementation of activities to enhance the quality of nursing practice
    - Participation on interdisciplinary teams that evaluate clinical practice or health services

2. The pediatric nurse uses the results of quality-of-care activities to initiate changes in practice.

3. The pediatric nurse uses the results of quality-of-care activities to initiate changes throughout the healthcare delivery system, as appropriate.

Additional Measurement Criteria for the Advanced Practice
Pediatric Nurse

4. The Advanced Practice Pediatric Nurse, as the clinical expert, assumes a leadership role in establishing and monitoring standards of practice to improve care of children and their families in collaboration with other healthcare team members.

5. The Advanced Practice Pediatric Nurse uses the results of quality-of-care activities to initiate changes throughout the healthcare system as appropriate.

6. The Advanced Practice Pediatric Nurse initiates interdisciplinary efforts to improve overall quality of care.

7. The Advanced Practice Pediatric Nurse participates in efforts to minimize costs and unnecessary duplication of tests and diagnostic services and facilitates the timely provision of services for the child and the family.

8. The Advanced Practice Pediatric Nurse analyzes factors related to safety, satisfaction, effectiveness, and cost/benefit options with the child and the family, and other healthcare providers as appropriate.

9. The Advanced Practice Pediatric Nurse analyzes organizational systems for barriers and promotes enhancements that affect child healthcare status.

10. The Advanced Practice Pediatric Nurse advocates for organizational, environmental, and practice changes to ensure that the unique needs of children are met during all aspects of their contact with the healthcare system.

11. Advanced Practice Pediatric Nurses base their evaluation of the quality of care on current knowledge, practice, and research.

Standard 2. Performance Appraisal

The pediatric nurse evaluates their own nursing practice in relation to professional practice standards and relevant statutes and regulations.

Measurement Criteria

1. The pediatric nurse engages in performance appraisal on a regular basis, identifying areas of strength as well as areas where professional development would be beneficial.

2. The pediatric nurse seeks constructive feedback regarding their own practice.

3. The pediatric nurse takes action to achieve goals identified during performance appraisal.

4. The pediatric nurse's practice reflects knowledge of current professional practice standards, laws, and regulations that affect the care of children and their families.

Additional Measurement Criteria for the Advanced Practice Pediatric Nurse

5. The Advanced Practice Pediatric Nurse engages in collaborative appraisal of professional practice with peers, patients, colleagues, and supervisors.

6. The Advanced Practice Pediatric Nurse has the inherent responsibility as a professional to evaluate their performance according to the standards of the profession, the standards specific to the specialty area, and various regulatory bodies, and to take action to improve practice.

7. The Advanced Practice Pediatric Nurse analyzes the effectiveness of interventions, the incidence and types of complications, and child outcome data to improve their own practice.

8. The Advanced Practice Pediatric Nurse takes action to achieve goals identified during performance appraisal and peer review, resulting in changes in practice and role performance.

Standard 3. Education

The pediatric nurse acquires and maintains current knowledge and competency in pediatric nursing practice.

Measurement Criteria

1. The pediatric nurse participates in ongoing nursing and interdisciplinary educational activities related to clinical knowledge and professional issues.

2. The pediatric nurse seeks childcare experiences that reflect current clinical practice in order to maintain current clinical skills and competence in the acute, outpatient, or home care settings.

3. The pediatric nurse acquires knowledge and skills appropriate to the care of children and their families and to the practice setting.

4. The pediatric nurse maintains knowledge of the developmental variances influencing children across the life cycle.

Additional Measurement Criteria for the Advanced Practice Pediatric Nurse

5. The Advanced Practice Pediatric Nurse uses current healthcare research to expand clinical knowledge, enhance role performance, and increase knowledge of professional issues.

6. The Advanced Practice Pediatric Nurse seeks experiences and formal and independent learning activities to maintain and develop clinical and professional skills and knowledge.

7. The Advanced Practice Pediatric Nurse seeks appropriate advanced practice certification when eligible.

Standard 4. Collegiality

The pediatric nurse interacts with, and contributes to, the professional development of peers, colleagues, and other healthcare providers.

Measurement Criteria

1. The pediatric nurse shares knowledge and skills with colleagues.

2. The pediatric nurse provides peers with constructive feedback regarding their practice.

3. The pediatric nurse interacts with colleagues to enhance their own professional nursing practice.

4. The pediatric nurse contributes to an environment that is conducive to the clinical education of nursing students, other healthcare students, and other employees, as appropriate.

5. The pediatric nurse contributes to a supportive and healthy work environment.

Additional Measurement Criteria for the Advanced Practice Pediatric Nurse

6. The Advanced Practice Pediatric Nurse contributes to the professional development of others to improve child health care and to foster the profession's growth.

7. The Advanced Practice Pediatric Nurse brings creativity and innovation to nursing practice to improve care delivery.

8. The Advanced Practice Pediatric Nurse serves as a leader for the purpose of influencing healthcare practice and policy for the care of children, families, and communities.

9. The Advanced Practice Pediatric Nurse participates in professional activities.

10. The Advanced Practice Pediatric Nurse contributes to an environment that is conducive to clinical education of other healthcare providers, including the acts of teaching, mentoring, and precepting, as appropriate.

Standard 5. Ethics

The pediatric nurse's assessment, actions, and recommendations on behalf of children and their families are determined in an ethical manner.

Measurement Criteria

1. The pediatric nurse's practice is guided by the *Code of Ethics for Nurses with Interpretive Statements*.[57]

2. The pediatric nurse maintains confidentiality within legal and regulatory parameters.

3. The pediatric nurse acts as an advocate for child and family care, and assists children and families in developing skills so they can advocate for themselves.

4. The pediatric nurse delivers care in a nonjudgmental and nondiscriminatory manner that is sensitive to children's and families' diversity.

5. The pediatric nurse delivers care in a manner that preserves and protects the child's and family's autonomy, dignity, and rights.

6. The pediatric nurse seeks available resources in formulating ethical decisions.

7. The pediatric nurse facilitates family participation in ethical decision-making.

8. The pediatric nurse offers or facilitates support for families making difficult ethical decisions.

9. The pediatric nurse works with families, social service agencies, and the courts when evidence exists for child abuse or neglect and other forms of family violence.

Additional Measurement Criteria for the Advanced Practice Pediatric Nurse

10. The Advanced Practice Pediatric Nurse ensures that the care provided is consistent with the patient's needs and values, and with *Code of Ethics for Nurses with Interpretive Statements*[57] and codes of ethical practice.

11. The Advanced Practice Pediatric Nurse makes decisions and initiates actions on behalf of children and their families in an ethical manner, taking into consideration the values of the child and the values of the family.

12. The Advanced Practice Pediatric Nurse maintains a therapeutic and professional relationship with the child and the family, and discusses the delineation of roles and parameters of the relationship with the child and the family.

13. The Advanced Practice Pediatric Nurse participates in obtaining the patient's informed consent or age-appropriate assent for procedures, treatment, and research, as appropriate.

14. The Advanced Practice Pediatric Nurse reports abuse of patients' rights and incompetent, unethical, or illegal practice.

15. The Advanced Practice Pediatric Nurse serves as an advocate for the child and the family in developing policy and in the provision of care services to the child and the family.

16. The Advanced Practice Pediatric Nurse contributes to the creation of individual and system responses to resolution of ethical dilemmas.

17. The Advanced Practice Pediatric Nurse advocates for a process of ongoing ethical inquiry into patient care practices where varying perspectives are acknowledged and validated.

Standard 6. Collaboration

The pediatric nurse collaborates with the child, family, and other healthcare providers in providing patient care.

Measurement Criteria

1. The pediatric nurse communicates with the child and family and other healthcare providers regarding the child's care and nursing's role in the provision of care.

2. The pediatric nurse collaborates with the child, family, and other appropriate healthcare providers in the formulation of overall goals and the plan of care, and in decisions related to care and the delivery of services.

3. The pediatric nurse consults with other healthcare providers for the child's and the family's care as needed.

4. The pediatric nurse makes referrals, including provisions for continuity of care, as needed.

5. The pediatric nurse assists the family in identifying and accessing community resources to support the family in the care of the child as appropriate.

*Additional Measurement Criteria for the Advanced Practice
Pediatric Nurse*

6. The Advanced Practice Pediatric Nurse consults with other
    healthcare providers to develop evidence-based protocols,
    standards, and guidelines for care.

7. The Advanced Practice Pediatric Nurse works with other
    disciplines to enhance care of the child and the family;
    interdisciplinary activities may include education, consultation,
    management, technological development, or research
    opportunities.

8. The Advanced Practice Pediatric Nurse facilitates an
    interdisciplinary process with other disciplines in teaching,
    consultation, management, and research activities, as
    appropriate.

Standard 7. Research

**The pediatric nurse contributes to nursing and pediatric health
care through the use of research methods and findings.**

Measurement Criteria

1. The pediatric nurse uses the best available evidence, preferably
    research data, to develop the plan of care and interventions.

2. The pediatric nurse participates in research activities as
    appropriate to the nurse's education, position, and practice
    environment. Such activities may include:

    -   Identifying clinical problems suitable for nursing research
    -   Participating in data collection
    -   Participating in a unit, organization, or community research
        committee or program
    -   Sharing research activities with others
    -   Conducting research
    -   Critiquing research for application to practice
    -   Using research findings in the development of policies,
        procedures, and practice guidelines for client care

3. The pediatric nurse participates in human subject protection activities as appropriate including age-appropriate, informed consent or assent for children who are under-age for informed consent.

Additional Measurement Criteria for the Advanced Practice Pediatric Nurse

4. The Advanced Practice Pediatric Nurse provides and supervises care that is substantiated by scientific evidence, as appropriate to the child's needs and the practice environment.

5. The Advanced Practice Pediatric Nurse critically evaluates existing practice in light of current and relevant research findings.

6. The Advanced Practice Pediatric Nurse identifies research questions in practice.

7. The Advanced Practice Pediatric Nurse adheres to family-centered research principles including:

   • Designing research that acknowledges the diversity of families, respecting their culture, ethnicity, values, priorities, and coping styles
   • Respecting the privacy and autonomy of families when conducting research
   • Providing families with complete and unbiased information about the purposes and uses of research and the possible benefits to children

8. The Advanced Practice Pediatric Nurse disseminates relevant research findings through practice, education, or consultation.

9. The Advanced Practice Pediatric Nurse ensures that children and families are supported in participating in research that is personally beneficial or meaningful to them.

Standard 8. Resource Utilization

The pediatric nurse considers factors related to safety, effectiveness, and cost in planning and delivering patient care.

Measurement Criteria

1. The pediatric nurse evaluates factors related to safety, effectiveness, availability, and cost when choosing between two or more practice options that would result in the same expected patient outcome.

2. The pediatric nurse assists the child and family in identifying and securing appropriate services available to address health-related needs.

3. The pediatric nurse assigns or delegates tasks as defined by the state Nurse Practice Acts and according to the knowledge and skills of the designated caregiver, which may include the child's family members.

4. If the nurse assigns or delegates tasks, it is based on the needs and condition of the child, the potential for harm, the stability of the child's condition, the complexity of the task, and the predictability of the outcome.

5. The pediatric nurse assists the child and family in becoming informed consumers about the costs, risks, and benefits of treatment and care.

6. The pediatric nurse assists the family in identifying and accessing resources for pediatric patients requiring long-term or rehabilitative care.

*Additional Measurement Criteria for the Advanced Practice
Pediatric Nurse*

7. The Advanced Practice Pediatric Nurse initiates ongoing activities to analyze patient care systems in an effort to improve the quality of care provided to children and their families.

8. The Advanced Practice Pediatric Nurse uses aggregate data, in cooperation with others, to develop or revise systems to avoid duplication of or gaps in service.

9. The Advanced Practice Pediatric Nurse advocates for the removal of barriers to care and for optimal care for the child and family.

GLOSSARY

Advanced Practice Pediatric Nurse (APPN). A licensed registered nurse (RN), educationally prepared at least at the master's degree level in the pediatric specialty, whose graduate level preparation is distinguished by a depth of knowledge of theory and practice, validated experience in clinical practice, and competence in advanced clinical nursing skills. The APPN focuses clinical practice on children, both healthy and those with acute or chronic conditions, and autonomously applies knowledge, skills, and experience to complex child health problems, with consideration given to the child within the context of the family system.

Assessment. A systematic, dynamic process by which the pediatric nurse, through interaction with the patient (or the patient's significant others) and healthcare providers, collects and analyzes data about the patient. Data may include the following dimensions: physical, psychological, sociocultural, spiritual, cognitive, functional, developmental, economic, and lifestyle.

Case management. A process of coordinating a child's healthcare services to achieve optimal quality care delivered in a cost-effective manner.

Certification. The formal process by which clinical competence is validated in an area of practice.

Child. A neonate (less than one month old, including those gestationally premature), infant, toddler, preschooler, or adolescent.

Continuity of care. An interdisciplinary process that includes the patient and patient's significant others in the development of a coordinated plan of care. This process facilitates the patient's transition between settings, based on changing needs and available resources.

Criteria. Relevant, measurable indicators of the standards of clinical nursing practice.

Diagnosis (diagnosing). *1.* The naming of the disease, illness, or syndrome a patient has or is believed to have, using classifications from various healthcare fields. *2.* A clinical judgment about the patient's response to actual or potential health conditions or needs, which provides the basis for determination of a plan of care to achieve expected outcomes. *3.* A clinical judgment to determine state of health, disease, illness, or injury, which depends upon the advanced synthesis of information obtained during the interview, physical exam, or diagnostic tests (e.g., lab, x-ray).

Differential diagnosis. The determination of which of two or more diseases or conditions with similar symptoms is most applicable, leaving only one disease or condition to which all symptoms point.

Evaluation. The process of determining both the client's progress toward the attainment of expected outcomes and the effectiveness of nursing care provided to the child and family.

Evidence-based. Founded on the collection, interpretation, and integration of valid, important, and applicable patient-reported, clinician-observed, and research-derived evidence. The best available evidence, moderated by patient circumstances and preferences, is applied to improve the quality of clinical judgments.[58]

Family. Family of origin or significant others as identified by the child or parents of the child.

Family-centered care. A philosophy of care that fully recognizes the vital role that the family plays in ensuring the health and well being of children, and acknowledges that emotional, social, and development support are integral components of child health care. This approach empowers families and fosters independence; supports family care-giving and decision-making; respects family choices; builds on family strengths; and involves families in all aspects of the planning, delivery, and evaluation of healthcare services. Information sharing and collaboration between families and staff are cornerstones of family-centered care.

Guidelines. The specification of a process of client care management which has the potential of improving the quality of clinical and consumer decision-making. Guidelines are systematically developed statements based on available scientific evidence and expert opinion.

Healthcare providers. Individuals with special expertise who provide healthcare services or assistance to children and their families. They may include nurses, physicians, psychologists, social workers, nutritionists, dietitians, child life specialists, and various therapists.

Implementation. May include any or all of the following activities: interviewing, delegating, and coordinating. The child, family, and healthcare providers may be designated to implement interventions within the plan of care.

Interventions. Nursing activities that promote and foster health, assess dysfunction, assist children to regain or improve their physical abilities, and prevent further disabilities. Nursing activities in child health care are aimed at both the child and the family.

Nurse. An individual who is licensed by a state agency to practice as a registered nurse.

Nurse Practice Act. State statute that defines the legal limits of practice for registered nurses.

Nursing. The diagnosis and treatment of human responses to actual or potential health problems.[2]

Nursing process. A systematic and interactive problem-solving approach that includes individualized patient and family assessment, planning, implementation/intervention, and evaluation.

Outcomes. Measurable, expected, family-centered goals that translate into observable behaviors.

Patient. Recipient of nursing care. The term *patient* is used in this document to provide consistency and brevity, bearing in mind that the terms *client, individual, child* or *family* might be better choices in some instances. When the patient is an individual child, the focus is on the health state, problems, or needs of a single person. When the patient is a family or group, the focus is on the well-being of the unit as a whole and the reciprocal effects of an individual's well-being on the other members of the unit. When the patient is a community, the focus is on personal and environmental health and the health risks facing certain specific population groups. Pediatric nursing practice recognizes that most often the recipient of care is both the individual child and the family because of the dependent relationship the child has with family members (particularly parents) and the legal responsibilities associated with the parenting role.

Pediatric nursing. Nursing practice which focuses on the care of children and their families within a variety of health care settings.

Plan of care. Comprehensive outline of care to be delivered to attain expected outcomes.

Prescriptive authority. The statutory or regulatory authority to prescribe drugs and devices as a component of a profession's scope of practice.

Quality of care. The degree to which health services for individuals and populations increase the likelihood of desired health outcomes and are consistent with current professional knowledge.

Recipients of pediatric nursing care. Children, groups, families, communities, or populations.

Registered Nurse (RN). An individual educationally prepared in nursing and licensed by the state board of nursing to practice nursing in that state. Registered nurses may be qualified for specialty practice at two levels—generalist and advanced. These levels are differentiated by educational preparation, professional experience, type of practice, and certification.

Significant others. Family members or those whom the family defines as persons who choose to be involved in care and care decisions.

Standard. Authoritative statement enunciated and promulgated by the profession, by which the quality of practice, service, or education can be judged.

Standards of care. Authoritative statements that describe a competent level of clinical nursing practice demonstrated through assessment, diagnosis, outcome identification, planning, implementation, and evaluation.

Standards of Nursing Practice. Authoritative statements that describe a level of care or performance common to the profession of nursing by which the quality of nursing practices can be judged. Standards of clinical nursing practice include both standards of care and standards of professional performance.

Standards of Professional Performance. Authoritative statements that describe a competent level of behavior in the professional role, including activities related to quality of care, performance appraisal, education, collegiality, ethics, collaboration, research, and resource utilization.

REFERENCES

1. American Nurses Association. 1996. *Scope and Standards of Advanced Practice Registered Nursing.* Washington, DC: American Nurses Association.

2. Kuntz, K. 1998. Working toward the future of pediatric advanced practice nursing. *Journal of the Society of Pediatric Nurses,* 3(2), 85–88.

3. American Nurses Association. 1995. *Nursing's Social Policy Statement.* Washington, DC: American Nurses Association.

4. Cronenwett, L. 1995. Molding the future of advanced practice nursing. *Nursing Outlook,* 43, 112–118.

5. American Nurses Association. 1998a. New scope of practice criteria approved. *The American Nurse,* p.26.

6. Pridham, K. 1995. *Standards and guidelines for pre-licensure and early professional education for the nursing care of children and their families.* Final report for Project # MCJ-559327, submitted to the Bureau of Maternal and Child Health (Title V, Social Security Act), Health Resources and Services, Bureau of Maternal and Child Health, Document #H112. Washington D.C.: U.S. Government Printing Office.

7. Woodring, B. (Ed.). 1998. *Standards and guidelines for pre-licensure and early professional education for the nursing care of children and their families.* Department of Health and Human Services, Bureau of Maternal and Child Health, Document #H112R77. Washington D.C.: U.S. Government Printing Office.

8. Kavanaugh, K. 1994. Family: Is there anything more diverse? *Pediatric Nursing,* 20(4), 423–426.

9. Family Service America. 1984. *The state of families, 1984–85.* New York: Family Service America.

10. Bozett, F. 1987. Family nursing and life-threatening illness. In M. Leahey & L. Wright(Eds.), *Families and Life-Threatening Illness* (pp. 2–25). Springhouse, PA: Springhouse.

11. Ahmann, E. 1994. Family-centered care: The time has come. *Pediatric Nursing*, 24(1), 52–53.

12. Shelton, T. L. Jeppson, E.S., & Johnson, B. H. 1987. *Family-Centered Care for Children with Special Heath Care Needs*. Washington, DC: Association for the Care of Children's Health.

13. Newacheck, P., & Stoddard, J. 1994. Prevalence and impact of multiple childhood chronic illnesses. *Journal of Pediatrics*, 124, 40–48.

14. Perrin, J., Guyer, B., & Lawrence, J.M. 1992. Health services for children and adolescents. *Future of Children*, 2(2), 25–39.

15. Burstein, K., & Bryan, T. 2000. Parents as partners in the medical home. *The Exceptional Parent*, 30(8), 29–31.

16. National Vital Statistics System. 2002. *America's Children: Key National Indicators of Well Being 2002*. Availiable at www.Childstats.gov/ac2002/highlight.asp

17. Annie Casey Foundation. 1999. *Kids Count Data Book*. Baltimore, MD.

18. Children's Defense Fund. 1998. *The State of America's Children*. Washington, DC: Children's Defenses Fund.

19. Brooten, D., Naylor, M., York, R., Brown, L., Roncoli, M., Hollingsworth, A., Cohen, S., Arnold, L., Finkler, S., Munro, B., & Jacobsen, B.1995. Effects of nurse specialist transitional care on patient outcomes and costs: Results of five randomized trials. *The American Journal of Managed Care*, 1, 45–51.

20. Brown, S. & Grimes, D. 1993. *Nurse Practitioners and Certified Nurse Midwives: A Meta-analysis of Studies on Nurses in Primary Care Roles*. Washington, DC: American Nurses Association.

21. O'Sullivan, A., L., & Jacobsen, B.S. 1992. A randomized trial of a health care program for first-time adolescent mothers and their infants. *Nursing Research*, 41(4), 210–215.

22. Safriet, B.J. 1992. Health care dollars and regulatory sense: The role of advanced practice nursing. *Yale Journal on Regulation*, 9(2), 417–488.

23. Thurber, F., & DiGiamarino, L. 1992. Development of a model of transitional care for the HIV-Positive child and family. *Clinical Nurse Specialist*, 6(3), 142–146.

24. Haber, J. 1997. Medicare reimbursement: A victory for APRNs. *American Journal of Nursing*, 11, 84.

25. Hamric, A., Spross, J., Hanson, C. 1996. *Advanced Nursing Practice: An Integrated Approach*. Philadelphia: W.B. Saunders.

26. National Council of State Boards of Nursing, Inc. 1993. *Draft: Model Nursing Administrative Rules for Advanced Nursing Practice*. Chicago, IL.

27. National Association of Pediatric Nurse Practitioners. 2002. *Scope of Practice Pediatric Nurse Practitioner in Primary Care*. Available at www. napnap.org

28. Division of Nursing, Bureau of Health Professionals, Health Resources and Services Administration. 1996. *The Registered Nurse Population. Findings from The National Sample Survey of Registered Nurses*. Rockville, MD: Division of Nursing.

29. Deatrick, J., Bartelone, C., Broome, M., Curley, M., Durand, B., Haack, M., Linden, L., Miles, M., Savedra, M., & Verger, J. 1998. Working towards the future of pediatric advanced practice nursing–part I. *Journal of the Society of Pediatric Nurses*, 3(2), 85–88.

30. Deatrick, J., Bartelone, C., Broome, M., Curley, M., Durand, B., Haack, M., Linden, L., Miles, M., Savedra, M., & Verger, J. 1999. Working towards the future of pediatric advanced practice nursing–part II. *Journal of the Society of Pediatric Nurses*, 4(1), 41–44.

31. U.S. Congress, Office of Technology Assessment. 1986. *Nurse Practitioners, Physician Assistants, and Certified Nurse Midwives. A policy analysis*. Washington, DC: US Government Printing Office.

32. Page, N., & Mackowiak, L. 1997. The clinical nurse specialist and nurse practitioner: Complementary roles. *Journal of the Society of Pediatric Nurses*, 2:4, 188–190.

33. Brundige, K. 1997. Preparing pediatric nurse practitioners for roles in specialty practice. *Journal of Pediatric Health Care*, 11, 198–200.

34. Aiken, L. & Salmon, M. 1994. Health care workforce priorities: What nursing should do now. *Inquiry*, 31, 318–319.

35. Reisinger, K., & Bires, J. 1980. Anticipatory guidance in pediatric practice. *Pediatrics*, 66, 889–892.

36. McEwen, M. 2003. *Community-based Nursing: An introduction (2nd Edition)*. Philadelphia: Saunders.

37. Madigan, E. 1997. An introduction to pediatric home health care. *Journal of the Society of Pediatric Nurses*, 2(4), 172–178.

38. Balinsky, W. 1999. Pediatric home care: Reimbursement and cost analysis. *Journal of Pediatric Health Care*, 13(6), 288–294.

39. Paladino, C. 2000. School nursing–scope of practice (part I). *New Jersey Nurse*, 30(9), 10–11.

40. Paladino, C. 2000. School nursing–scope of practice (part II). *New Jersey Nurse*, 30(10), 3, 6.

41. Wann, M. 1994. Flight nurses find job satisfaction in the air. *Nurseweek*, 7(14), 1, 8, 21.

42. Reiser, J. 1998. Flight nursing: The National Flight Nurses Association—past, present, and future. *Journal of Emergency Nursing*, 24(6), 571–573.

43. Air and Surface Transport Nurses Association. 2002. *Transport Nurse FAQ's*. Available at www.astna.org

44. Solomon, M. 1998. Camp nursing: Rising to the challenge. *NurseWeek*, 11(11), 26–27.

45. Feeg, V. 1989. A unique setting for pediatrics: The hole in the wall gang camp. *Pediatric Nursing*, 15(4), 329–332.

46. Selekman, J. 1995. Standards and guidelines for pediatric prelicensure nursing education published. *Pediatric Nursing*, 21(6), 541–542.

47. Selekman, J., & Woodring, B. 2002. The changing dynamics of pediatric pre-licensure education. *Pediatric Nursing*, 28(4), 367–371.

48. National Organization of Nurse Practitioner Faculties. 1995. *Advanced Nursing Practice: Curriculum Guidelines and Program Standards for Nurse Practitioner Education*. Washington, DC: NONPF.

49. American College of Nurse-Midwives. 2002. *Core Competencies for Basic Mid-wifery Practice*. Washington, DC: ACNM.

50. American Association of Nurse Anesthetists. 1999. *Standards for Accreditation of Nurse Anesthetists Educational Programs*. Park Ridge, IL: AANA.

51. American Nurses Association and Society of Pediatric Nurses. 1996. *Statement on the Scope and Standards of Pediatric Clinical Nursing Practice*. Washington, DC: ANA/SPN.

52. Association of Faculties of Pediatric Nurse Practitioners and Associate Programs. 1996. *Philosophy, Conceptual Model, Terminal Competencies for the Pediatric Nurse Practitioner*. Washington, DC: AFPNPAP.

53. American Nurses Credentialing Center. 2002. *Certification Catalog*. Washington, D.C. American Nurses Credentialing Center.

54. Bowden, V. 1999. Certification opportunities for pediatric nurses. *Pediatric Nursing*, 25(5), 547–554.

55. Lyon, B. 1997. News from the National Association of Clinical Nurse Specialists, *Clinical Nurse Specialist*, 6, 235.

56. American Nurses Association. 1998. *Standards of Clinical Nursing Practice (2nd Edition)*. Kansas City, MO: American Nurses Association.

57. American Nurses Association. 2001. *Code of Ethics for Nurses with Interpretive Statements*. Kansas City, MO: American Nurses Association

58. McKibbon, K.A., Wilczynski, N., Hayward, R.S., Walker-Dilks, C.J., & Hayes, R.B. 1995. The medical literature as a resource for evidence based practice. Working Paper from the Health Information Research Unit, McMaster University, Ontario, Canada.

59. American Association of Colleges of Nursing. 1990. *A Database for Graduate Education in Nursing, Summary Report.* Washington, DC: AACN.

60. American Association of Colleges of Nursing. 1996. *The Essentials of Master's Education for Advanced Practice Nursing.* Washington, DC: AACN.

61. National Task Force on Quality Nurse Practitioner Education. 2002. *Criteria for Evaluation of Nurse Practitioner Programs: Report of the National Task Force on Quality Nurse Practitioner Education.* Washington, DC: National Task Force.

62. American Academy of Nurse Practitioners. 2003. *Position Statement on Nurse Practitioner Curriculum.* Austin, TX: Author. Available at www.aanp.org

63. National Certification Board of Pediatric Practitioners and Nurses. 2003. *Pediatric Nurse Practitioner Certification and Certification Maintenance Programs.* Gaithersburg, MD: Author. Available at www. pnpcert.org.

64. Lewandowski, L.A., & Tesler, M.D. 2003. *Family-Centered Care: Putting it into Action—The SPN/ANA Guide to Family-Centered Care.* Washington, DC: nursebooks.org.

Appendix

Guidelines for
Advanced Practice Pediatric
Registered Nurse Education

Background

Post-baccalaureate education for professional practice has become the norm for many healthcare providers. Physicians and pharmacists have identified such needs and established educational criteria accordingly. Allied health colleagues, such as social workers, physical therapists, and nutritionists, have more recently increased the educational requirements for entry into professional practice to include a minimum of a master's degree.

Although consensus has not been obtained on the educational level required for entry into nursing practice, consensus has been reached related to the educational level needed to enter advanced practice nursing. Practitioners and educators alike agree that a master's degree in nursing is the minimal acceptable educational credential for the Advanced Practice Registered Nurse (APRN). Thus, while master's preparation in nursing has existed since the 1950s, the degree is now the educational foundation for all APRNs.

According to the data provided by the American Association of Colleges of Nursing (AACN),[59] masters' level nursing programs have widely divergent clinical practice requirements, didactic course experiences, and end-product titling. The curricula of some graduate programs do not include direct patient and family care experiences and provide little exposure to concepts related to advancing the profession. These findings led the AACN to develop *The Essentials of Master's Education for Advanced Practice Nursing.*[60] This seminal document clearly identifies the foundation upon which any advanced practice program should be built. Likewise, the National Organization of Nurse Practitioner Faculties (NONPF),[48] the National

Task Force on Quality Nurse Practitioner Education,[61] the American Academy of Nurse Practitioners (AANP),[62] the Association of Faculties of Pediatric Nurse Practitioners and Associate Programs (AFPNP/AP),[52] and the National Certification Board of Pediatric Nurse Practitioners and Nurses (NCBPNP/N)[63] provide standards, guidelines, and competencies for nurse practitioner programs.

AACN conceptualized the three components of all APRN master's curricula: graduate nursing core, advanced practice nursing core, and specialty curriculum content. Specialty organizations were directed to develop guidelines for specialty-specific content. The purpose of this appendix is to describe specialty-specific content within the overall curriculum common to all pediatric APRNs and to compare the content with practice standards. Guidelines for pre-licensure education were developed in collaboration with the Bureau of Maternal and Child Health;[6-7] however, none previously existed for pediatric APRN education.

Education and Practice

Standards of practice describe professionally authorized aspects of the care process and professional performance, while guidelines for education describe suggested areas of curricular focus for the APRN master's level nursing programs (see Table 1).

Course Work and Clinical Experience

The course work and clinical experience in the advance practice pediatric curriculum are consistent with that developed by the AACN. Both are designed to enable graduates of advanced practice pediatric programs to attain the standard of care as outlined in the *Statement on the Scope and Standards of Pediatric Clinical Nursing Practice*.[51]

Course work generic to all master's level nursing curricula includes content in the following areas: theoretical foundations of nursing practice, (evaluation) research, evidence-based practice, policy, organization, and financing of health care, ethics, professional role skills and development, and human diversity. Course work with a pediatric focus includes content in advanced health and physical assessment, genetics, advanced physiology and pathophysiology,

Table 1: *Comparison of Standards of Advanced Pediatric Practice Registered Nursing and Guidelines for Advanced Nursing Education*

Standards of Advanced Pediatric Practice Registered Nursing	Guidelines for Advanced Pediatric Practice Nursing Education
Standards of Care	*Areas of Curricular Focus*
1. Assessment	Advanced health and physical assessment, advanced physiology and pathophysiology, genetics, advanced child and family development, family theories
2. Diagnosis	Clinical decision-making
3. Outcome identification	Clinical decision-making
4. Planning	Clinical decision-making
5. Implementation	
5a. Coordination of comprehensive health services	Family-centered care
5b. Consultation	Professional role skills and development
5c. Health promotion, health maintenance, and health teaching	Promotion, maintenance, and (re) habilitation of optimal health with well children, acutely ill, seriously ill, and critically ill children Management of acute and chronic conditions
5d. Prescriptive authority	Advanced pharmacology
5e. Referral	Clinical decision-making
6. Evaluation	(Evaluation) research
Standards of Professional Performance	*Areas of Curricular Focus*
1. Quality of care	(Evaluation) research
2. Performance appraisal	Professional role skills and development
3. Education	Professional role skills and development
4. Collegiality	Policy, organization, and financing of health care
5. Ethics	Ethics, human diversity
6. Collaboration	Professional role skills and development
7. Research	Theoretical foundations of nursing practice Research
8. Resource utilization	Evidence-based practice

family theories, advanced pharmacology, advanced child and family development, clinical decision-making, family-centered care, promotion, maintenance, and (re) habilitation of optimal health with well children, acutely ill, seriously ill, and critically ill children, and management of acute and chronic conditions.

Clinical practice experiences in diverse settings are a vital part of the curriculum. Clinical experiences may focus on the care of children in clinics, in-patient units, homes, and a variety of community settings including school-based clinics and day care centers. Clinical experience builds on course work and is designed to enable graduates of advanced pediatric programs to collect health data, establish a diagnosis, identify expected outcomes individualized to the child and family, plan and prescribe care, implement interventions, and evaluate the child's and family's progress toward attainment of outcomes. Opportunity is provided for students to work collaboratively in the context of an interdisciplinary team. The goals of all clinical experiences are the opportunity to develop and to apply technical skills, critical thinking, theory, leadership, and research in the care of children and their families, and to work as an integral part of the healthcare team. Specific competencies are outlined in areas of curricular focus in the section to follow. Of course, enactment of these competencies is influenced by the practice context and by health policy and regulation on the organizational, state, and federal levels.

Faculty

Ideally, academic faculty responsible for the overall implementation of advanced practice programs should be prepared at the doctoral level and be actively engaged in practice settings with children and their families as educators, researchers, or clinicians. Teams of faculty should be involved in the development, implementation, and evaluation of the advanced practice education program. A complement of individual faculty with diverse backgrounds and expertise in research and practice is necessary to provide students with a broad education that will prepare them to deal with future challenges in health care. Faculty are ultimately responsible for the students' learning and clinical experiences related to children and families within or outside of the hospital setting. It is essential that faculty be academically prepared as well as competent in their area of teaching. The minimum educational credential for faculty is a master's degree in nursing.

Clinical preceptors play a critical role in the evolution of the Advanced Practice Pediatric Nurse; therefore, preceptors will ideally be master's prepared nurses who have demonstrated outstanding clinical expertise in a field related to pediatric advanced practice. The preceptor must also be knowledgeable in the areas of teaching and educational evaluation. If a preceptor does not possess these latter educational skills, it becomes incumbent upon the academic educator to assist the preceptor in attaining them. A collaborative relationship between the academic educator and the preceptor is necessary for fostering optimal learning experiences for the students. The academic educator must be able to interpret the clinical objectives and outcome criteria to the preceptor and assist the preceptor in selecting appropriate patient-focused learning activities when needed.

Areas of Curricular Focus and Competencies

Course work and clinical experiences during graduate study will provide the APRN with knowledge and skills enabling the demonstration of beginning competencies in the following areas:

1.   Pediatric Advanced Physiology and Pathophysiology

2.   Genetics

3.   Advanced Pharmacology

4.   Advanced Child And Family Development

5.   Pediatric Advanced Health and Physical Assessment

   • Uses multifaceted assessment strategies for monitoring and evaluating the needs of individual children and their families and in planning programs for aggregates of children and their families.

   • Provides anticipatory guidance to children and their families for expected and potential changes regarding child and family health.

6. Clinical Decision-Making
   Demonstrates critical thinking and diagnostic reasoning skills in clinical decision-making regarding children's health.

7. Promotion, Maintenance, and (Re) Habilitation of Optimal Health With Well, Acutely Ill, Seriously Ill, and Critically Ill Children

8. Management of Acute and Chronic Conditions
   - Manages rapidly changing situations regarding the health care of children.
   - Assists others in decision-making in rapidly changing situations.
   - Assists children and their families to integrate implications of their illness, recovery, and long-term wellness into their lifestyles.
   - Assists children and their families to alter lifestyles to meet changing developmental and healthcare needs.
   - Teaches and empowers children's self care and development of responsibility for care.
   - Assists children and their families with goal setting for health promotion and maintenance.

9. Family-Centered Care
   - Ensures comprehensive family-centered care through collaboration with the family and the healthcare providers.
   - Creates a relationship that acknowledges and supports strengths, coping strategies, and development of children and their families to address healthcare needs to the extent possible.
   - Protects and enhances the individual worth of every child within the context of family-centered care.
   - Recognizes, detects, and attends to expressed and unexpressed meanings, feelings, and concerns.
   - Recognizes and monitors own emotional response to the children's and family's behaviors, using this awareness to facilitate therapeutic interaction.
   - Provides comfort or communication through touch as appropriate.
   - Provides emotional and informational support to children and their families.

- Counsels children and their families in crisis or suffering grief, and refers as appropriate.
- Assists children and their families with participation in care and decision-making, including problem solving with clinicians.
- Negotiates an agreement when priorities of the children, families, and providers conflict.

10. Professional Role Skills And Development
    - Functions in a variety of role dimensions: consultant, educator, supervisor, administrator, researcher, and clinician within a variety of settings serving children and their families.
    - Interprets own professional strengths, role, and scope of practice to children, families, and colleagues.
    - Participates in self-evaluation and the review of other health practitioners. Continuously updates knowledge base and clinical competencies regarding care of children and their families as well as areas of special expertise.
    - Meets and maintains eligibility requirements for certification.
    - Communicates the children's health status using appropriate format and technology.
    - Collaborates with the multidisciplinary healthcare team to support the process of health promotion and to achieve maximal wellness for children and their families.
    - Gives constructive feedback to other healthcare providers to ensure safe care practices.
    - Confronts inappropriate healthcare practices by peers, colleagues, caregivers, and family members in the care of children and their families.
    - Interprets and promotes the Advanced Practice Pediatric Nurse role to the public and other healthcare professions.
    - Supports socialization, education, and training of novice Advanced Practice Pediatric Nurses by serving as preceptor, role model, and mentor.

11. Consultation
    Consults with children, families, providers, healthcare systems, and communities regarding child healthcare issues.

12. Teaching
    - Teaches children, families, providers, healthcare systems, and communities regarding child healthcare issues.
    - Promotes an environment that facilitates learning.
    - Identifies readiness to learn.
    - Assesses health behaviors, care-related issues and tasks, and learning needs of children and their families.
    - Assesses barriers to health behavior change by children and their families.
    - Establishes plans and standards for group and individual teaching.
    - Provides anticipatory guidance appropriate for age and developmental status.
    - Develops an understanding of illness and disease that supports adaptive functioning and participation in care.
    - Provides explanations of treatment in developmentally appropriate language.
    - Provides information about therapeutic actions, side effects, and instructions to promote participation and optimum wellness for children and their families.
    - Develops educational programs appropriate to optimal wellness and health problems, level of functioning and understanding, emotional needs, and individual characteristics.

13. Directing Care
    - Uses discretionary judgment in assessing conflicting priorities and needs.
    - Builds and maintains a therapeutic team to provide optimum therapy. Manages selected aspects of organizational function (e.g., staff, budget, computer systems, interpersonal relationships, access to services, and other resources).
    - Collaborates with case managers and case specialists caring for children and their families.
    - Acts as case manager, advocating for the needs of children and their families.

14. Providing Leadership
    - Maintains active membership in professional organizations.
    - Provides leadership in professional activities at the local, state, and national levels.

15. Policy, Organization, and Financing of Health Care
    - Demonstrates knowledge of the healthcare environment.
    - Evaluates implications of contemporary health policy for children, families, healthcare providers, communities, and states, as well as the nation and the world.
    - Participates in legislative and policy-making activities influencing health and social services practices which affect children and their families.
    - Assists children and their families in accessing appropriate healthcare resources.

16. Ethics

17. Human Diversity
    - Develops a system of personal ethics in professional practice within the context of children and family issues, based on ethical principles and codes.
    - Provides culturally competent care for children and their families.

18. Theoretical Foundations of Nursing Practice

19. Child and Family Theories
    Practices from a framework of theories and concepts from nursing, and critiques and applies theories from basic and other applied sciences.

20. (Evaluation) Research

21. Evidence-Based Practice
    - Participates in, and uses results of, clinical research in the management of children and families with a variety of healthcare needs.
    - Selects and recommends appropriate nursing interventions for children and their families with attention to safety, cost, invasiveness, acceptability, and efficacy.

- Incorporates professional and legal standards into practice with children and their families.
- Identifies the need for a systemic study.
- Critically evaluates and applies research studies pertinent to the management of children's health care.
- Uses the continuous quality improvement process to examine the efficacy and acceptability of care for children and their families.
- Monitors quality of own practice.
- Maintains comprehensive database for ongoing evaluation of own practice.
- Indicates evaluation of care through follow-up, consultation, peer review, and other means.
- Uses knowledge of therapeutic regimens and children and family responses for evaluation of care.
- Engages in research use, dissemination, and knowledge generation for the care of children and their families.
- Participates in organized efforts to develop performance measures and implement guidelines.

INDEX

An index entry preceded by a bracketed calendar year indicates an entry from a previous edition or predecessor publication that is included in this edition as an appendix. Thus, [2004] is *Scope and Standards of Pediatric Nursing Practice* (Appendix A) and [2003] is *Standards of Cardiovascular Nursing Practice* (Appendix B).

A

Accountability, 2, 6, 19, 34, 118, 119
  [2004] 88
Acute care pediatric nurse practitioner
  (PNPAC), 18
Acute care in pediatric nursing, 22
Advanced practice pediatric nursing,
  9
  [2003] 104–110, 121
  advocacy, 75
  assessment, 42
  [2003] 129, 163
  collaboration, 65
  [2003] 146
  collegiality, 64
  [2003] 143
  consultation, 53
  [2003] 135, 163
  coordination of care, 50
  [2003] 134, 163
  defined, [2003] 149
  diagnosis, 43
  [2003] 130, 163
  education, 30, 63
  [2003] 109, 116–117, 142, 161–170
  ethics, 66–67
  [2003] 144–145
  evaluation, 56–57
  [2003] 138
  health teaching and health promotion,
    51–52
  [2003] 136, 163
  implementation, 48–49
  [2003] 134, 163
  leadership, 72–73
  [2003] 169
  outcomes identification, 44–45

  [2003] 131, 163
  planning, 47
  [2003] 132–133, 163
  prescriptive authority and treatment,
    21, 54
  [2003] 136–137, 163
  professional practice evaluation, 62
  [2003] 141
  quality of practice, 60
  [2003] 140
  referral, 55
  [2003] 137, 163
  research, 69
  [2003] 147
  resource utilization, 70–71
  [2003] 148
  roles, 18–22
  [2003] 109
  work environment, 3
  See also Acute care pediatric nurse
    practitioner (PNPAC); Neonatal
    nurse practitioner (NNP); Pediatric
    clinical nurse specialist (PCNS);
    Primary care pediatric nurse
    practitioner (PNP-PC)
Advanced practice registered nurse
  (APRN), 18
  [2003] 101, 104, 149, 161
Advocacy, 32, 36–37
  ethics and, 35
  standard of professional performance,
    6, 74–75
Age-appropriate care. *See* Cultural
  competence and competencies
Ambulatory care, 23
American Nurses Association (ANA), *xi*,
  1, 2

American Nurses Credentialing Center
(ANCC), 19, 33–34
  [2003] 118
Analysis. *See* Critical thinking, analysis,
  and synthesis
Assessment
  [2003] 163, 165
  [2004] 86–87
  defined, [2003] 149
  diagnosis and, 43
  [2003] 129–130
  evaluation and, [2003] 138
  standard of practice, 39–42
  [2003] 127–129
Assumptions of pediatric nursing
  practice, 3
  [2003] 120

B
Body of knowledge
  education and, 32–33
  [2003] 117–118
  professional practice evaluation,
  [2003] 167
  See also Evidence-based practice

C
Camp care, 26–27
  [2003] 115–116
Care recipients. *See* Patients
Care standards. *See* Standards of
  practice
Case management, 11, 50
  [2003] 134, 149
  See also Coordination of care
Certification and credentialing, 25,
  32–33
  [2003] 117–118, 149, 165–170
  [2004] 88
*Changes in Healthcare Professions'
  Scope of Practice: Legislative
  Consideration, xii*
Child, [2003] 100–101, 149
Clients. *See* Patients
Clinical nurse specialist (CNS). *See*
  Pediatric clinical nurse specialist
  (PCNS)

Clinical settings. *See* Practice settings
*Code of Ethics for Nurses with Interpretive
  Statements,* 1
  See also Ethics
Collaboration, 15, 29, 60
  [2003] 99
  [2004] 87–88
  implementation and, 48
  standard of professional performance,
  65
  [2003] 145–146, 163, 166
  See also Healthcare providers; Interdisciplinary health care
Collegiality
  standard of professional performance,
  64
  [2003] 142–143
Communication, 15, 17
  [2003] 99
Community health care, 24–26
  [2003] 112
Competence assessment. *See*
  Certification and credentialing
Complementary therapies, 28–29
Confidentiality. *See* Ethics
Consultation
  standard of practice, 53
  [2003] 135, 163, 167
Continuity of care, [2003] 149
Coordination of care, 11, 50
  leadership and, [2003] 168
  standard of practice, 50
  [2003] 134, 149, 163
  See also Interdisciplinary health care
Cost control
  coordination of care and, 50
  outcomes identification and, [2003]
  130–131
  quality of practice and, 59–60
  resource utilization and, 70–71
Cost-effectiveness. *See* Cost control
Credentialing. *See* Certification and
  credentialing
Criteria. *See* Measurement criteria
Critical thinking, analysis, and synthesis,
  18
  [2003] 166

Crossing the Quality Chasm: A New Health System for the 21st Century, 16
Cultural competence and competencies, 9–10, 15
[2003] 99, 149, 169
in standards of nursing practice, 4, 27

D
Data collection, 68
[2003] 146
assessment and, 39
[2003] 127–129
Data and pediatric nursing practice. *See* Data collection
Decision-making
[2003] 166–167
consultation and, 52–53
ethics and, 66
[2003] 109, 144
leadership and, 72
Diagnosis
[2003] 109, 163
[2004] 87
defined, [2003] 150
standard of practice, 43
[2003] 129–130
Differential diagnosis, [2003] 130, 150
Diversity issues. *See* Cultural competence and competencies
Documentation
evaluation and, 57
professional practice evaluation and, 61
Domains and Core Competencies of Nurse Practitioner Practice, 1

E
Economic issues. *See* Cost control
Education of patients and families
[2003] 111
See also Families; Health teaching and health promotion; Patients
Education of pediatric nurses, 29–32
[2003] 116–117, 142
[2004] 86
collegiality and, 64
credentialing and, 18
curriculum guidelines, [2003] 161–170

leadership and, [2003] 106
standard of professional performance, 63
See also Mentoring; Professional development
Environment. *See* Practice environment
Ethics, 35–36
[2003] 169
standard of professional performance, 66–67
[2003] 143–145
See also Code of Ethics for Nurses with Interpretive Statements; Laws, statutes, and regulations
Evaluation
[2003] 169
[2004] 87
defined, [2003] 150
health teaching and health promotion, 51
standard of practice, 56–57
[2003] 138
Evidence-based practice, 6–7, 14–16
[2003] 150, 169–170
assessment and, 39–40
implementation and, 15–16, 18
outcomes identification and, 44
standard of professional performance, 68–69
See also Research

F
Families
[2003] 150
assessment and, [2003] 165–166
collaboration, [2003] 168
collaboration and, 15
coordination of care, [2003] 166–167
coordination of care and, 3–4
See also Education of patients and families; Patients
Family-centered care, 1
[2003] 150–151, 166–167
defined, 13–14
[2003] 97–98
elements, 14, 15
[2003] 98–99

Family-centered care (*continued*)
  SPN/ANA Guide, 14
Financial issues. *See* Cost control

G
Generalist practice pediatric nursing,
    17–18, 29–30
  [2003] 103–104, 116
  See also Pediatric nursing
Guidelines, 7, 11–14
  [2003] 124, 151, 162–170

H
Healthcare policy, [2003] 169
Healthcare providers
  [2003] 151
  assessment and, 39
  coordination of care and, 50
  diagnosis and, 43
  outcomes identification and, 44
  See also Collaboration; Inter-
    disciplinary health care
Healthcare team. *See* Collaboration;
    Interdisciplinary health care
Health teaching and health promotion
  [2003] 111, 163
  standard of practice, 51–52
  [2003] 136, 168
*Healthy Eating and Activity Together
  (HEAT) obesity prevention
  (NAPNAP),* 16
Home care, 11–13
  [2003] 112–113
Hospice care, 23
Human resources. *See* Professional
    development

I
Implementation
  consultation, 53
  [2003] 163
  coordination of care and, 50
  [2003] 163
  defined, [2003] 151
  evaluation and, 56
  health teaching and health promotion,
    [2003] 163

planning and, 46
prescriptive authority and treatment,
    [2003] 163
quality of care and, [2003] 139
referral, [2003] 163
standard of practice, 48–49
  [2003] 133–134
Information. *See* Data collection
Inpatient care, 22
  [2003] 110–111
Institute of Medicine (IOM), *Crossing
    the Quality Chasm,* 16
Interdisciplinary health care
  underlying assumptions, *xii*
  quality of care and, [2003] 139
  See also Collaboration; Healthcare
    providers
*International Classification of
    Functioning, Disability and Health-
    Children and Youth Version (ICF-
    CY),* 3
Interventions
  [2003] 151
  [2004] 87

K
Knowledge base. *See* Body of knowledge
*KySSM: Keep Your Children/Yourself Safe
    and Secure,* programs (NAPNAP),16

L
Laws, statutes, and regulations, 33–34
  [2003] 118
  professional practice evaluation and,
    61
  [2003] 141
  See also Ethics
Leadership
  [2003] 169
  standard of professional performance,
    72–73
Levels of practice. *See* Advanced
    practice pediatric nursing;
    Generalist practice pediatric
    nursing
Licensing. *See* Certification and
    credentialing

M
Measurement criteria in pediatric
  nursing, 7
  [2003] 123–124, 150
  advocacy, 74–75
  assessment, 39–42
  [2003] 127–129
  collaboration, 65
  [2003] 145–146
  collegiality, 64
  [2003] 142–143
  consultation, 53
  [2003] 135
  coordination of care, 50
  [2003] 134
  diagnosis, 43
  [2003] 129–130
  education, 63
  [2003] 142
  ethics, 66–67
  [2003] 143–145
  evaluation, 56–57
  [2003] 138
  health teaching and health promotion,
  51–52
  [2003] 136
  implementation, 48–49
  [2003] 133–134
  leadership, 72–73
  outcomes identification, 44–45
  [2003] 130–131
  planning, 46–47
  [2003] 132–133
  prescriptive authority and treatment,
  54
  [2003] 136–137
  professional practice evaluation, 61–
  62
  [2003] 141
  quality of practice, 59–60
  [2003] 139–140
  referral, 55
  [2003] 137
  research, 68–69
  [2003] 146–147
  resource utilization, 70–71
  [2003] 148

Mentoring
  collegiality, [2003] 143
  collegiality and, 64
  leadership and, 72
Multidisciplinary healthcare. See Interdisciplinary health care

N
National Association of Pediatric Nurse
  Practitioners (NAPNAP)
  about, *v, xii–xiii*
  definition of pediatric population, 1
  definition of pediatric nurse
  practitioner (PNP), [2003] 107
  prevention programs, 16
  Scope and Standards of Practice:
  Pediatric Nurse Practitioner (PNP),
  xii, 2
Nurse, [2003] 151
Nurse Practice Act, [2003] 151
Nurse practitioner (NP). *See* Neonatal
  nurse practitioner (NNP); Pediatric
  nurse practitioner (PNP)
Nursing: Scope and Standards of Practice,
  1
Nursing, [2003] 151
Nursing Excellence for Children and
  Families, 11
Nursing process, 5–6
  [2003] 151
  See also Standards of practice
Nursing's Social Policy Statement, 1
Nursing standards. *See* Standards of
  practice; Standards of professional
  performance

O
Organizations. *See* Professional
  organizations in nursing
Outcomes
  [2003] 163
  collaboration and, 65
  defined, [2003] 152
  diagnosis and, 43
  ethics and, 66
  evaluation and, 56
  planning and, 46–47

Outcomes (*continued*)
  quality of practice and, 59–60
  resource utilization and, 70–71
  standard of practice, 44–45
  See also Outcomes identification
Outcomes identification
  standard of practice, 44–45
  [2003] 130–131
  See also Outcomes
Outpatient care, [2003] 111–112

P
Palliative care, 23
Parents. *See* Families
Patients
  [2003] 152
  coordination of care and, 3–4
  ethics, [2003] 145
  ethics and, 66
  See also Education of patients and
    families; Families
Pediatric clinical nurse specialist
    (PCNS), 18–19, 30–31
  [2003] 106
Pediatric nurse practitioner (PNP), 19–21,
    31
  [2003] 106–108
  [2004] 86–88
  acute care pediatric nurse practitioner
    (PNPAC), 20–21
  primary care pediatric nurse
    practitioner (PNP-PC), 19–20
Pediatric nursing
  certification, 32–33
  competencies, 17–18
  complementary therapies, 28–29
  cultural competencies, 9–10
  defined, [2003] 152
  education, 29–32
  focus on family, 1
  global perspectives, 28
  history and development, *xi-xiii*
  interdisciplinary assumption, *xii*
  levels of practice, [2003] 103–110
  practice context, 9–11
  roles, 18
  [2003] 106–108

scope of practice
  [2003] 103–110
  [2004] 86
settings for, 22–27
  [2003] 110–116
standards of practice, 39–57
  [2003] 127–138
  [2004] 86–88
standards of professional performance,
    59–75
  [2003] 139–148
  See also Advanced practice pediatric
    nursing; Scope of practice of
    pediatric nursing; Standards of
    practice for pediatric nursing;
    Standards of professional
    performance for pediatric nursing
Pediatric population, definition of, 1
Peer review and relations (nurse). *See
  also* Accountability; Performance
  appraisal
Performance appraisal, [2003] 141
Perioperative care, 22
Plan of care, [2003] 152
Planning
  [2003] 163
  resource utilization and, 70
  [2003] 148
  standard of practice, 46–47
  [2003] 132–133
Policy. *See* Healthcare policy
Practice environments, 22–27
  [2003] 100–101, 110–116
Practice roles. *See* Roles in pediatric
  nursing practice
Practice settings. *See* Practice
  environments
Preceptors. *See* Mentoring
Prescriptive authority and treatment
  [2003] 152
  standard of practice, 54
  [2003] 136–137, 163
Primary care pediatric nurse practitioner
    (PNP-PC), 18
Privacy. *See* Confidentiality
Professional development, 8
  collegiality and, 64
  [2003] 142

professional practice evaluation and, 61
  [2003] 141
  See also Education; Leadership
Professional issues and trends, 34–35
Professional organizations in nursing, *v*,
  33
  American Nurses Association, *xi*, 1, 2
  certification, [2003] 117–118
  See also , National Association of
    Pediatric Nurse Practitioners
    (NAPNAP); Society of Pediatric
    Nurses (SPN)
Professional performance. *See*
  Standards of professional
  performance
Professional practice evaluation,
  standard of professional
  performance, 61–62

Q
Quality of practice, 11–14
  [2003] 152
  [2004] 88
  standard of professional performance,
    59–60
  [2003] 139–140

R
Recipients of care. *See* Patients
Recipients of pediatric nursing care,
  [2003] 152
Referral
  standard of practice, 55
  [2003] 137, 163
  See also Collaboration; Coordination
    of care
Registered nurse (RN)
  [2003] 153
  See also Advanced practice registered
    nurse (APRN)
Regulatory issues. *See* Laws, statutes,
  and regulations; Laws, statutes and
  regulations
Research
  [2003] 169
  assessment and, 42
  [2003] 129

education and, 63
  [2003] 142
  planning and, 46, 47
  [2003] 132
  standard of professional performance,
    68–69
  [2003] 146–147
  See also Evidence-based practice
Resource, standard of professional
  performance, 70–71
Resource utilization
  standard of professional performance,
    70–71
  [2003] 148
Roles in pediatric nursing practice, 18
  [2003] 106–108
  See also Advanced practice pediatric
    nursing; Nursing role specialty;
    Pediatric clinical nurse specialist;
    Pediatric nurse practitioner

S
Safety assurance, 17
  [2003] 104
School-centered care, 24–26
  [2003] 113–114
Scientific findings. *See* Evidence-based
  practice; Research
Scope of practice of pediatric nursing,
  xi, 2
  [2003] 103–110
  [2004; PNP] 86
Self care and self-management, [2003]
  166
Settings. *See* Practice environments
Significant others
  [2003] 153
  See also Families
Society of Pediatric Nurses (SPN)
  about, *v, xii*
  established Advanced Practice Task
    Force, [2003] 92, 104
  *Scope and Standards of Pediatric
    Nursing Practice, ix*, 2
  *SPN/ANA Guide to Family-Centered
    Care*, 14
  [2003] 98

Society of Pediatric Nurses (*continued*)
    Statement on the Scope and Standard
        of Pediatric Clinical Nursing Practice,
    [2003] 93
Specialty certification. *See* Certification
    and credentialing
Standard (defined), 2
    [2003] 153
Standards of care for pediatric nursing
    [2003] 122–123
    defined, [2003] 153
    origins, [2003] 92–93
    See also Standards of practice for
        pediatric nursing
Standards of practice for pediatric
        nursing, 4–5
    [2003] 119, 153
    assessment, 39–42
        [2003] 127–129, 163
        [2004] 86–87
    assumptions, 3
        [2003] 120
    consultation, 53
        [2003] 135, 163
    coordination of care, 50
        [2003] 134, 163
    development, 2
        [2003] 119
    diagnosis, 43
        [2003] 129–130, 163
        [2004] 86–87
    evaluation, 56–57
        [2003] 138
        [2004] 87
    health teaching and health promotion,
        51–52
        [2003] 136, 163
    implementation, 48–49
        [2003] 133–134, 163
    organizing principles, 3–4
        [2003] 120–122
    outcomes identification, 44–45
        [2003] 130–131, 163
    planning, 46–47
        [2003] 132–133, 163
    prescriptive authority and treatment, 54
        [2003] 136–137, 163

referral, 55
    [2003] 137, 163
themes, 6
    [2003] 122–123
    See also each standard
Standards of professional performance
        for pediatric nursing, 6–7
    [2003] 123, 153
    advocacy, 74–75
    collaboration, 65
        [2003] 145–146, 163
        [2004] 87–88
    collegiality, 64
        [2003] 142–143, 163
    education, 63
        [2003] 142, 163
    ethics, 66–67
        [2003] 143–145, 163
    leadership, 6, 72–73
    performance appraisal, [2003] 163
    professional practice evaluation, 61–62
        [2003] 141
    quality of practice, 59–60
        [2003] 139, 163
        [2004] 88
    research, 6, 68–69
        [2003] 146–147, 163
    resource utilization, 70–71
        [2003] 148, 163
    See also each standard
Surgical care, 22
Synthesis. *See* Critical thinking, analysis,
    and synthesis

T
Teaching. *See* Education; Health teaching
    and health promotion
Teams and teamwork. *See*
    Interdisciplinary health care
Terminology, [2003] 149–153
Transport care, 26
    [2003] 114–115
Trends in pediatric nursing practice, 34–35

W
Work environments. *See* Practice
    environments